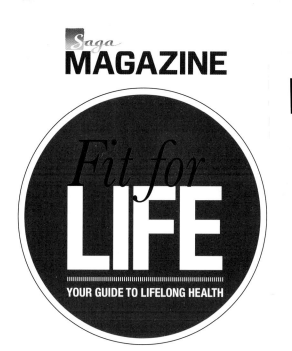

Saga MAGAZINE

Fit for LIFE
YOUR GUIDE TO LIFELONG HEALTH

Editor Sarah Russell
Contributors Evie Serventi, Kate Percy
Art Director Jo Gurney
Sub Editor Rachel Storry
Advertising Director Katie Wood (020 7907 6689)
Advertising Account manager Simone Daws (020 7907 6617)
Photography Dana Patrick, Danny Bird, Fotolia
Model Jo Price

With thanks to Katy Bravery and her staff for their expertise, the Physical Company (www.physicalcompany.co.uk) and Brooks (www.brooksrunning.co.uk) for providing equipment and clothing for our photo shoots

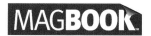

DENNIS PUBLISHING LTD
MagBook Publisher • **Dharmesh Mistry**
MagBook Manager • **Tommy Melville**
Digital Production Manager • **Nicky Baker**
Operations Director • **Robin Ryan**
MD of advertising • **Julian Lloyd-Evans**
Newstrade Director • **David Barker**
MD of Enterprise • **Martin Belson**
Chief Operating Officer • **Brett Reynolds**
Group Finance Director • **Ian Leggett**
Chief Executive • **James Tye**
Chairman • **Felix Dennis**

LICENSING AND SYNDICATION
To license this product please contact Carlotta Serantoni on +44 (0) 20 79076550 or email carlotta_serantoni@dennis.co.uk
To syndicate content from this product please contact Anj Dosaj Halai on +44(0) 20 7907 6132 or email anj_dosaj-halai@dennis.co.uk

The MagBook brand is a trademark of Dennis Publishing Ltd., 30 Cleveland St, London W1T 4JD. Company registered in England. All material © Dennis Publishing Ltd, licensed by Felden 2013, and may not be reproduced in whole or part without the consent of the publishers.

Fit for Life: Your Guide to Lifelong Health
ISBN 1-78106-263-3

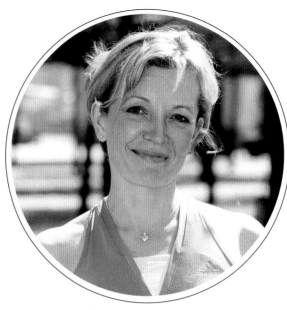

WELCOME...

Welcome to *Fit for Life*! I'm absolutely delighted that you've picked up this exciting, new publication and that you're interested in improving your health, fitness and wellbeing.

Thanks to new research and medical developments, our life expectancy continues to rise, and most of us will reach our 80s or beyond. But living longer is only part of the story. We don't just want to age, we want to do it with vitality, mobility, good health, fitness and a passion to live life to the full.

Our goal with *Fit for Life* was to create an innovative publication, packed full of statistics, snippets of information, expert comments, research, ideas, and motivation on almost every topic of health, fitness and nutrition you can think of.

We've tried to feature some of the most relevant issues that we face as we get older. We've covered everything from bowel cancer to beetroot juice, magnesium to menopause and Alzheimer's to avocados. There may be

topics that you're already familiar with, and there may be things that surprise you. We hope that you'll find it interesting, motivating and educational, and have a few "I never knew that!" moments as you're reading through.

I've worked in the health and fitness industry for over 20 years; as a journalist, coach, personal trainer and health expert. And, over that time, I've seen the recommendations on health and fitness change constantly, as experts uncover more about the human body and how to stay healthy, avoid disease and live longer.

It can be hard to keep up with this pace of change, and even harder to adjust our habits of a lifetime. But adopt an open mindset, a positive "can do" attitude and take responsibility for your own health, and you'll be well on the way to being "Fit for Life".

Sarah Russell

Fit for LIFE
Contributors

Editor Sarah Russell

Sarah Russell has over 20 years' experience in the fitness industry as a running coach, trainer, freelance writer, weight management coach and athlete. She also has a Masters degree in Sport Science, and is a qualified England Athletics Running Coach and Biomechanics Coach. She is a competitive runner and triathlete, having completed nine marathons and various long-distance triathlons, representing Great Britain in the duathlon. Former Editor of *Fitness for Women*, she has written for various publications, including *Running Fitness, Bodyfit, Women's Weekly, Weightwatchers, Running Free* and *Nuffield Health,* and was the Chief Contributor of *The Ultimate Guide to Marathon Running*. She balances her time between writing, training runners and biomechanics coaching. *www.sarah-russell.co.uk*

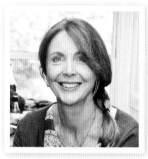

Contributor Kate Percy

Athlete, cook and food for fitness writer, Kate Percy offers top healthy eating advice and puts it into practice with delicious recipes for active people. Kate's books *Go Faster Food* and *Go Faster Food for Kids* are available on *amazon.co.uk,* at *www.gofasterfood.com* and in all good bookstores. She's also written for the *Sunday Times, Runner's World, Running Fitness, 220 Triathlon, Cycling Plus, Health & Fitness Magazine, Women's Running, Men's Health, FHM* and other fitness magazines.

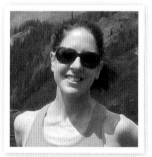

Chief Contributor Evie Serventi

Evie is an Australian journalist and editor who has lived and worked in the UK for the past five years. She is a dedicated runner, and freelance editor and writer in the health and fitness industry. She's passionate about mental performance and motivation, which complements her current post-graduate studies in psychology, and she loves to help people achieve their goals and improve their performance. *www.evieserventi.com* Evie tweets @hotoffthepage

Contents

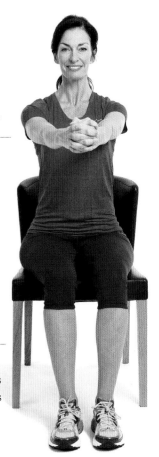

Know it

If you love your sport or exercise, you will probably be very conscious of maintaining your health and if you really give it your all, you may well need to provide your body with greater levels of nutritional support.

Nexgen® has been formulated for those undertaking regular training or exercise with the highest quality chelated minerals for superior absorption. With a total of 28 ingredients including magnesium, natural vitamin K2-MK7, vitamin D3 and a range of micronutrients including DeltaGold® delta-tocotrienols, Lyc-O-Mato® (natural lycopene), BIOLUT™ lutein esters, grapeseed extract, green tea extract, Selenium SeLECT® and natural coenzyme Q10.

This spectrum of ingredients contributes to normal muscle function, a reduction of tiredness and fatigue, normal energy-yielding metabolism and normal protein synthesis, the normal function of the immune system and the maintenance of normal bones. It also contributes to normal absorption of calcium and phosphorous as well as normal blood calcium levels.

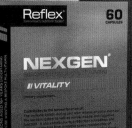

£9.59

www.reflex-nutrition.com

Reflex®
Tomorrow's nutrition today™

'Take care of your body; it's the only place you have to live'

Jim Rohn

Health

Over the next few pages, you'll find information on some of the most relevant health topics that face us as we get older; in particular, the most common concerns for people over the age of 50

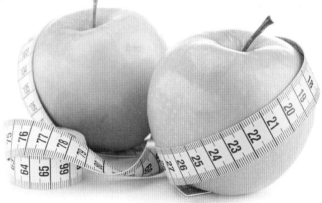

You may be familiar with some of the conditions, possibly even have one yourself or know a friend or family member who is affected. Others will be news to you, and the facts and figures may surprise or shock you.

'Whilst some of the statistics may make for uncomfortable reading, knowing the facts is vital and could well save your life. Our mission with this book is to raise awareness of the most important health concerns facing our society today, the symptoms of various conditions and, most importantly, what you can do to reduce your risk of getting them in the first place.

It may be tempting to skip this section. It's normal to feel uncomfortable when we talk about cancer, bowel health and other embarrassing conditions. But we urge you to read and absorb the information, especially about the symptoms. You never know when you might need it.

But what can we do about it?

Prevention is always better than cure, and there's a lot we can all do to avoid illness, disease and various health conditions, especially cancer. Our modern-day lifestyle, however, doesn't make it easy.

We're faced with junk food and oversized portions at every turn. We lead busy, but often sedentary, lives centred around computers, televisions and labour saving devices. Most of us are stressed, even those who are retired, and we don't get enough sleep or exercise.Most alarming of all is that 61% of the UK population is now overweight or obese.

Being healthy in our current society means challenging the status quo. It might not always be easy, but we must actively choose to make healthier and more informed decisions about what we eat, how we move and our lifestyle choices.

We hope that this book will provide you with up-to-date facts and figures, some ideas and, most of all, some motivation to take good care of yourself.

Eat well, move more and take control of your health. After all, no-one else will do it for you.

Heart disease

Coronary heart disease is still the most common cause of death in the UK, so make sure you're aware of the symptoms and don't ignore them, no matter how mild

There are many different types of heart conditions and problems, including angina, heart attacks, heart failure and abnormal heart rhythms. The most common problem is known as coronary heart disease (CHD), where your arteries become narrowed by a build-up known as atherosclerosis. This can result in angina or a heart attack.

There are around 2.3 million people living with CHD in the UK, and around 80,000 people die from CHD every year. Even though this figure has halved since 1961, CHD is still the most common cause of death in the UK in 2013.

Causes and prevention

Risk factors include being overweight, having diabetes, smoking, drinking, high blood pressure, high blood cholesterol and stress, as well as having a family history of heart disease, especially in a relative under the age of 55. The more risk factors you have, the greater your chance of developing CHD. You can significantly reduce your risk by making changes to your lifestyle. Ask your GP for a heart health check, and ask them for support to help you make changes, or check out the NHS Change 4 Life programme at *www.nhs.uk/change4life*.

Symptoms

Symptoms of a heart attack may include chest pain or discomfort, which can also spread to your arm, neck, jaw, stomach or back; a dull pain, ache or heavy feeling in your chest; a feeling of indigestion, which can make you feel quite unwell; and feeling sick, sweaty, breathless, dizzy or generally unwell.

> ## *Did you know?*
>
> **Physical activity is one of the most important things you can do to reduce your risk of developing heart disease. According to the British Heart Foundation Physical Activity Statistics 2012, 20–35% of cardiovascular diseases could be prevented if more people become more active throughout the life course. Exercise needs to be regular (30 minutes five times per week) and aerobic, where you get your heart rate up and feel slightly out of breath. Brisk walking, jogging, cycling and dancing are all great.**

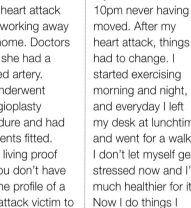

Maureen's Story

Maureen Hennis, 65, had a heart attack in 2012

Maureen suffered a major heart attack when working away from home. Doctors found she had a blocked artery. She underwent an angioplasty procedure and had two stents fitted.

"I'm living proof that you don't have to fit the profile of a heart attack victim to have heart problems. I was healthy, fit and a non-smoker, but I was also an absolute workaholic. Some days I could be at my desk from 7am to 10pm never having moved. After my heart attack, things had to change. I started exercising morning and night, and everyday I left my desk at lunchtime and went for a walk. I don't let myself get stressed now and I'm much healthier for it. Now I do things I never thought I'd do before my heart attack. I'm living a healthy, happier and more relaxed life!"

WITH THANKS TO THE BRITISH HEART FOUNDATION: WWW.BHF.ORG.UK

Our expert says

"Aspirin can help in an emergency. If you think you're having a heart attack, the most important thing to do is call 999 and then sit and rest while you wait for the ambulance. But if you have some to hand, and you're not allergic, you should also chew an adult aspirin."

Amy Thompson, Senior Cardiac Nurse at the British Heart Foundation

WHAT TO DO...

Symptoms can vary greatly so don't ignore them. They can be mild or severe, but in all cases phone 999 for an ambulance if you have any of the symptoms of a heart attack. Don't worry about bothering the ambulance crew or doctors; if you think it might be a heart attack, it's always better to dial 999.

Angina can feel like a heaviness or tightness in your chest and can spread to your arms, neck, jaw and stomach, too. Some people have a shortness of breath or describe their discomfort as a dull ache. It's often brought on by exercise, stress, cold weather or after eating. Symptoms of angina tend to subside after a few minutes but if you think you might be suffering from angina, see your doctor as soon as possible. CHD isn't reversible, but you can prevent it from worsening by keeping a heart healthy and with medical treatment.

Stroke

There are over 152,000 strokes in the UK each year. One in five is fatal, and stroke remains the main cause of severe adult disability and the third largest cause of death behind heart disease and cancer

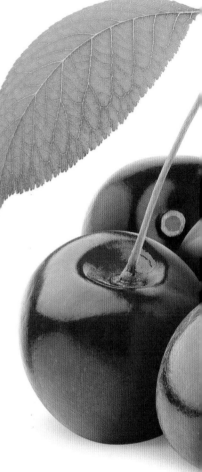

People over 65 are at more risk of having a stroke, but younger people, including children and even babies, can have them, too. Strokes affect people in different ways, depending on the part of the brain that's affected and how severe the damage is, but the healthier and fitter you are the more you reduce your risks of having a stroke in the first place.

Symptoms

Stroke is always a medical emergency, so time really is crucial in terms of recognising the symptoms and taking appropriate action. Although signs and symptoms vary for everyone, it's worth learning the FAST test to recognise symptoms of a stroke or mini-stroke (transient ischaemic attack, or TIA):

Facial weakness: has the person's face drooped (usually down one side)?

Arm weakness: is the person able to lift both arms above their head?

Speech problems: does the person's speech sound slurred?

Time to call 999: if one or more of these symptoms are present, call 999 immediately.

The FAST test identifies stroke nine times out of ten.

Aside from treating a TIA as a serious warning sign, dizziness, sudden loss of vision, problems with balance and coordination, and difficulty swallowing can also be symptoms of a stroke. Other rarer and more subtle symptoms include sudden, severe headache; sudden memory loss or confusion; and loss of or blurred vision.

Causes and prevention

Maintaining a healthy lifestyle helps to lower your risk of having a stroke. Keep your weight down, avoid smoking and watch your alcohol intake; eat a healthy diet and exercise regularly. Have regular health checks to monitor your blood pressure and cholesterol.

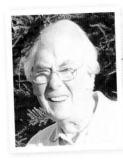

Tony's Story

Tony, 78, from Leicester, had a TIA in February 2011.

Tony's son was visiting when he noticed his dad's face had dropped on one side. It only lasted for ten minutes, and Tony felt fine afterwards.

During a regular check-up about a week later, Tony mentioned it to his GP, who referred him to the stroke centre straightaway. A brain scan showed that he'd had a TIA, and he was put on medication.

Being proactive essentially prevented Tony from having a full stroke, and he concurs that anyone experiencing any FAST symptoms should go straight to their local stroke centre, as the sooner you get there the more they can do for you.

Tony, who says he feels healthy for his age, now maintains his fitness with tennis, bowling, badminton and daily walks.

With thanks to The Stroke Association: www.stroke.org.uk

Our expert says

"Stroke devastates lives, but many can be prevented. Everyone can reduce their risk by making simple lifestyle changes, like stopping smoking, eating a healthy, balanced diet and exercising regularly. High-blood pressure (hypertension) is the single biggest risk factor and causes over half of all strokes and TIAs. It's really important to get your blood pressure checked regularly, and if it's high you can take steps to regulate it."
*Dr Peter Coleman,
Deputy Director of Research for the
Stroke Association*

WHAT TO DO...

If you think you or someone near you is experiencing one or more FAST symptoms, call 999 immediately. Symptoms of a TIA last from minutes to a few hours before disappearing, so it's key to see your GP as soon as possible if you think you've had a TIA. If a TIA is identified, you'll receive further tests and a brain scan to decide how to lower your risk of stroke.

Depression

Depression is a physical illness that can impact both your mind and your body. It's fairly common in the UK, with around 15% of people over the age of 65 having symptoms of depression

According to new research from the English Longitudinal Study of Ageing (ELSA), at the University College of London, people over 50 who are physically active generally live longer and have better mental health.

Symptoms

Symptoms can be physical (changes in appetite or sex drive, sleep problems, low energy, aches and pains); behavioural (avoiding people and social events, agitation, feeling demotivated); emotional (hopelessness, feeling anxious and/or constantly unhappy); and, in severe cases, psychotic (delusions, hallucinations, feeling suicidal).

We all get sad and go through ups and downs, but if you feel any depressive symptoms intensely or persistently for weeks or months it's time to be proactive and seek help. If

SEEKING SUPPORT
Age UK Advice:
0800 169 65 65
www.ageuk.org.uk
Mind: 0300 123 3393
www.mind.org.uk
Depression Alliance:
0845 123 23 20 www.
depressionalliance.org

you're concerned a relative or friend might have symptoms of depression, try talking to them about it. Watch for signs of self-neglect and drinking more alcohol. Encourage them to see their GP and offer to go along.

Causes and prevention

While depression can develop out of the blue, it's often triggered by a significant event such as losing a loved one, losing your job, semi-retiring/ change of daily routine, or coping with a long-term injury

or chronic health condition. Poor physical health is one of the most common risk factors contributing to depression as you get older. Others include money worries, excessive alcohol and not feeling needed. The hormonal changes women go through during the menopause can also affect their emotional and mental wellbeing.

Anticipate events that might add extra stress or pressure to your life, and seek support and help early on. Socialising and social networking can help you feel connected and part of your local community. Keep active, as there's evidence that regular exercise and being in nature through hobbies such as gardening and yoga help keep your mood even, your mind calm and your coping skills sharp.

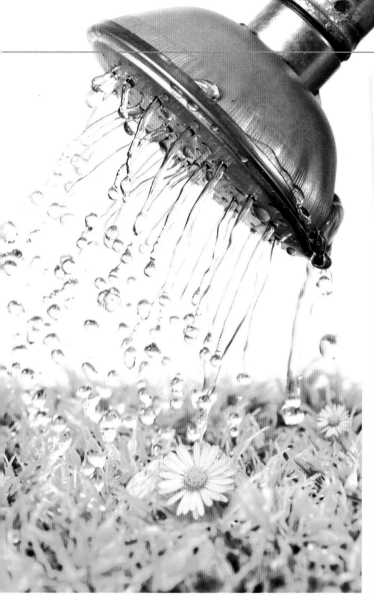

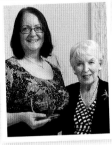

Jan's story

Jan Tchamani, 56, lives in Birmingham with her husband

"Life throws curve balls at you, but it's important to realise this usually means it's offering up new opportunities. I believe that if you're suffering in your mind over a long period, it's often a sign your lifestyle needs radical adjustments. When a friend at work recognised I was having a breakdown, I was referred to occupational health for an assessment. I was diagnosed with rapid cycling bipolar (a lifelong condition) around my 50th birthday.

"As well as professional intervention, such as medication and talking therapies, and support from organisations such as Bipolar UK and Mind, I believe spending time in nature, a creative activity like writing, healthy eating and exercise play an important role in self-management. I find a smörgåsbord of strategies to be the best, combined with excellent self-knowledge, and an awareness of triggers and warning signs. My earliest warning signs were physical: shivery shoulders, the world around me losing its colours and flavours, feeling sleepy...

"Finding like-minded people in your area by joining a micro community such as a gardening group is a good connection to make. I'm finding that community food growing is bringing people together in an inspiring way. And gardening is a slowed-down activity that helps you focus on a simple outcome and takes your mind off your problems."

CASE STUDY IMAGE: JUNE WHITFIELD PRESENTING JAN WITH THE 'AGE UK INTERNET CHAMPION OF THE YEAR 2013'. WWW.AGEUK.ORG.UK/INTERNET-CHAMPIONS. WITH THANKS TO AGE UK: WWW.AGEUK.ORG.UK BRITISH PSYCHOLOGY SOCIETY: WWW.BPS.ORG.UK, MIND: WWW.MIND.ORG.UK

WHAT TO DO...

See your GP before you reach a tipping point to discuss how you're feeling if you think you might be depressed, as this alone may lift your spirits. Your GP will assess you, and talk through things that might be contributing to how you're feeling. If diagnosed with depression, depending on how mild or severe your condition is, your GP will advise you about the next step. Talking treatments (therapies) are free to those on the NHS, whether you're diagnosed with depression or just feel lonely and need someone to talk to.

Stress

In the UK, one in five people live with very high levels of anxiety. What's more worrying, 84% of GPs are seeing more patients for stress and anxiety issues than ever before

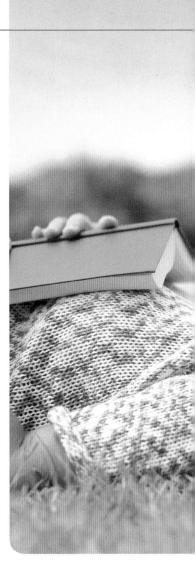

What are the symptoms?

"Hurry sickness" (always being in a hurry), putting yourself under pressure even when it's not necessary, non-specific hostility, feeling angry, feeling threatened by life's demands and by other people, sleeplessness, difficulty getting to sleep, or waking in the early hours, feeling the joy has gone out of life, resistance to change, even impaired memory.

Physical symptoms include: excessive sweating and tension, inability to relax, palpitations or racing heartbeat, digestive disorders such as irritable bowel syndrome (IBS), and relying increasingly on alcohol, or other mood-altering substances.

Causes and prevention

"Try not to get into a worked-up state about

Did you know?

Both laughter and owning a pet are great ways to relieve stress. Studies show that unconditional love from a pet can reduce tension and boost your mood; and laughter has been shown to reduce the level of stress hormones, boost endorphin levels and even increase your immunity.

situations that really aren't life threatening," says Psychotherapist Susan Balfour, author of *Stress Control: Stress-Busting Strategies for the 21st Century.* "Tension in the muscles signals 'danger' to the brain, which in turn switches on the fight or flight response – this response is essential in the face of a real emergency,

but harmful when triggered for situations that do not require running away from danger.

"The stress response raises blood pressure, produces excess sugar and fats, shuts down the digestive system, reduces sexual libido and can cause panic attacks," says Balfour.

Learning to slow down and relax is essential. Practise positive thinking, and try doing

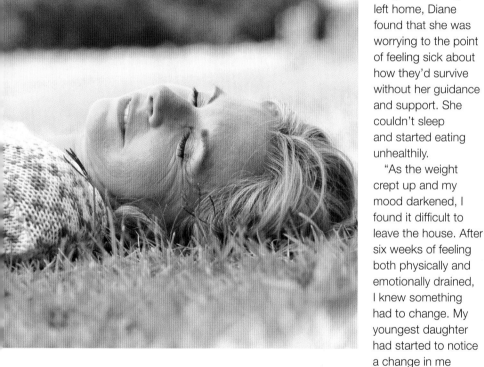

Diane's story

Diane, 57, lives in Cardiff with her husband

With all three of her daughters having left home, Diane found that she was worrying to the point of feeling sick about how they'd survive without her guidance and support. She couldn't sleep and started eating unhealthily.

"As the weight crept up and my mood darkened, I found it difficult to leave the house. After six weeks of feeling both physically and emotionally drained, I knew something had to change. My youngest daughter had started to notice a change in me when we spoke on the phone, and my relationship with my husband was deteriorating. I was so caught up in my own despair that I'd forgotten about the ones around me who I loved."

Diane started taking a vitamin (Super Once A Day, from Quest Vitamins), began sleeping better and had more energy. "Once the tiredness was under control, I felt more positive. I started to exercise – taking the dog on long walks and going swimming – which not only did wonders for my figure but for my whole mental attitude. I still worry about my children, but I've learned not to let that worry spiral out of control."

With thanks to CCD PR: www.ccdpr.com

yoga or "mindfulness training", giving full attention to the present moment. Get adequate sleep and exercise regularly. Avoid excessive amounts of alcohol, tobacco and junk food such as crisps, cake and processed snacks.

Our expert says

"One of the greatest threats is ignoring stress. As life gets busier, people tend to pile more onto their plate. Yet we all need space to relax, whether through hobbies, socialising with friends or exercising. This helps you maintain a sound perspective of your life and allows you to take a step back and see things clearly. The most important thing is to take it seriously and to identify ways to help you de-stress."
Peter Karataos, Consultant Clinical Psychologist

WHAT TO DO...

Start keeping a diary of your stress episodes, and if you feel the same after two weeks see your GP to discuss your symptoms and referral options, such as a stress management group, cognitive behavioural therapy (CBT) or other talking therapies.

Menopause

The menopause is known as the 'change of life' or when menstruation stops. The average age for women in the UK to reach menopause is 52 and if it occurs under 45, it is known as premature menopause

Menopausal symptoms affect about 70% of women and are the main reason women take hormone replacement therapy (HRT). While symptoms are usually linked to hormonal changes and the natural drop in oestrogen; diet, exercise, lifestyle and other medication can also influence your symptoms'

Symptoms

Perimenopausal symptoms include hot flushes, night sweats, mood swings, palpitations, insomnia, joint aches and vaginal dryness. The hot flush (or flash) affects around 60-85% of menopausal women.

Later menopausal symptoms include: discomfort on passing urine; passing urine more often during the day/night; urine infection; leakage of urine; and vaginal dryness, discomfort, discharge, burning and itching.

Did you know?

As a natural alternative to HRT, Promensil Red Clover Isoflavones have been clinically proven to help reduce hot flushes and night sweats by up to 73%: www.promensil.co.uk

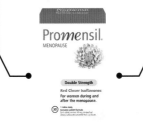

Causes and prevention

A natural phase of life, the menopause is caused by a change in the balance of the body's sex hormones. Hormonal changes affect every woman differently, and adopting a healthy lifestyle and maintaining a good diet can help you mitigate menopausal symptoms. Avoid smoking, as women who smoke typically have an earlier menopause and perimenopause than women who don't. And avoid caffeine and alcohol, which can make flushes worse. Exercise 30 minutes, five times a week.

Our expert says

"As far as health is concerned, I encourage women to acknowledge that a natural menopause often marks a point in mid-life when women can work towards maintaining a healthy weight, taking regular exercise and making healthy lifestyle choices, such as not smoking and moderating alcohol intake. Making these changes will improve health at the time of the menopause and lead to improved future health."
Kathy Abernethy, Senior Nurse Specialist, Menopause Clinical and Research Unit, Northwick Park Hospital, Harrow

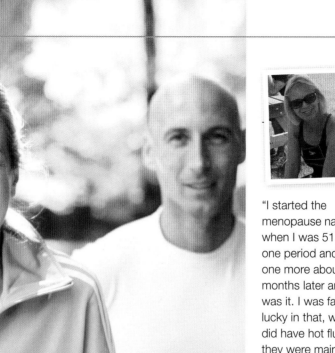

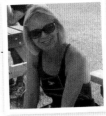

Tanya's Story

Tanya, 59, lives in Surrey with her husband

"I started the menopause naturally when I was 51. I had one period and then one more about six months later and that was it. I was fairly lucky in that, while I did have hot flushes, they were mainly at night and I could almost time them to the minute! I also felt achier all over. These symptoms continued on and off for a few years, but never really effected my life.

"I think exercise helped with the whole experience. I've always been sporty, and when I was going through the change exercising helped keep my mood even and spirits up. Some of my friends had other symptoms such as getting teary and mood swings, yet my symptoms seemed mild in comparison.

"If you factor fitness into your daily routine, it becomes a part of everyday life. Every week I swim two or three times, play tennis once and run or cycle twice. I don't push myself to the extreme; I just do what I enjoy and what feels right, and that includes eating a healthy diet"

WHAT TO DO...

See your GP if you're experiencing symptoms that are disrupting your quality of life. There's no specific test to diagnose the menopause, but a blood test to measure the level of follicle-stimulating hormone might be recommended. HRT is one of the main treatments for the menopause. It's available in many forms: creams, tablets, gel, a skin patch or an implant.

Before seeing your GP, think about family history, and read up on symptoms and other management options such as homeopathic remedies, acupuncture and herbal remedies. Think about how you might make positive changes to your lifestyle, diet and fitness regime. Arming yourself with knowledge and self-awareness will make your GP visit more effective.

Dementia

There are about 800,000 people in the UK with dementia, including one in 14 people over the age of 65. Alzheimer's disease affects around 496,000 people in the UK and is the most common cause of dementia

There's no known cure for Alzheimer's and sadly it's progressive. The good news, however, is that you can reduce the risk of developing Alzheimer's through healthy living and addressing lifestyle factors such as smoking, obesity, diabetes, high blood pressure and high cholesterol.

In a nutshell, be stubborn about maintaining a healthy lifestyle, and you'll improve your chances of being "head strong" in later life.

Symptoms

Early on, you may experience memory lapses and struggle to find the right words. As the disease progresses, you may become confused and frequently forget the names of people, places, appointments and recent events. You may have mood swings and feel sad, angry or afraid over increasing memory loss. Increased confusion and difficulty with everyday activities are common symptoms.

Did you know?

Exercise has been linked with preventing the development of Alzheimer's and improving mild cognitive function in new research published in the *Journal of Alzheimer's Disease*. The study monitored two groups of 66 to 88-year-olds on a 12-week exercise programme.

Causes and prevention

Age is the main factor affecting Alzheimer's and, once you reach 65, the chances of developing the condition doubles every five years. Genetic factors are also relevant: in rare cases, Alzheimer's is caused by the inheritance of a single gene, increasing the risks of developing the condition.

Maintain a healthy and balanced diet, exercise regularly and avoid smoking. Exercising for 30 minutes at least five times a week helps with weight management and can help reduce the risk of developing Alzheimer's.

Our expert says

"New management options for Alzheimer's disease are

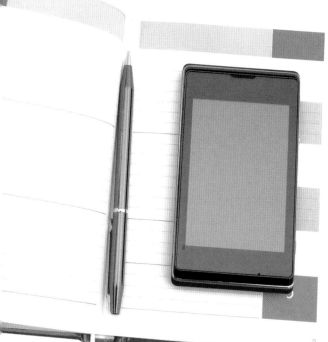

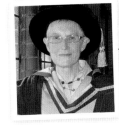

Ann's Story

Ann Johnson, 59, was diagnosed with Alzheimer's disease when she was 52

"People are scared of the word dementia, but they just need to understand they have a condition and learn how to deal with it. I'm a great advocate of early diagnosis. If you find your memory loss is getting worse and causing you problems, go and talk to your GP promptly.

"There are three things that keep me going: friends, faith and doing my talks. I go out every day for a walk. I try not to think too far ahead; I just go from day to day with the help of good friends."

Ann's tips:
"Write lists! Use a dictaphone to record future tasks and events. I have to decide where my limitations are; if I know I can't do something, I have to accept it."

Ann raises awareness of dementia with the Alzheimer's Society and received an Order of the British Empire for her inspiring work.

being explored all the time, with a recent focus on lifestyle approaches. Ensure any signs of high blood pressure or heart disease are treated, ensure weight is controlled and diabetes excluded or managed properly, and undertake regular physical exercise. A diet rich in antioxidants and specific nutrients that help the brain replace cell membranes needed to maintain nerve cell function are important, too; and some nutritional supplements such as Souvenaid and other dietary supplements like flavonoids are being used more widely."
Dr David Wilkinson, Consultant in Old Age Psychiatry, Memory Assessment and Research Centre, Moorgreen Hospital

B vitamins

Growing research suggests B vitamins can help protect the parts of the brain affected by Alzheimer's. Boost B12 oral spray from BetterYou is in the form of Methylcobalamin, the form that's naturally present in our bodies and therefore the most readily absorbed: *www.betteryou. uk.com*

WHAT TO DO...

If your memory is getting worse and impacting on your daily life, see your GP. Watch out for regular confusion; forgetting the names of friends or objects; and forgetting things you've heard, seen or read.

The Alzheimer's Society provides information and support, as well as dementia cafés, where people can chat about living with dementia.
***www.alzheimers.org.uk*; National Dementia Helpline: 0300 222 1122**

Sleep

Quality sleep is vital for our health and wellbeing, but according to a recent report four out of five people in the UK complain of disturbed or inadequate sleep

Sleep is a basic human need, yet many of us underestimate the importance of not only the amount of sleep we get, but also the quality. We need sleep to help us function normally, and inadequate sleep over a period of time can leave us in sleep debt. This can have a negative effect on our thinking and mood, and can lead to long-term health problems.

A major report recently published by The Sleep Council (*www.sleepcouncil.org.uk*) has shown that 47% of people in the UK say that stress or worry keeps them awake at night and are too anxious to sleep. The same report also highlights a worrying number of people surviving on only five to six hours' sleep per night. While the amount of sleep we need varies from person to person, recommendations suggest a minimum of six to nine hours per night to feel refreshed.

Top tips for great sleep

Top tips from Dr Jason Ellis, leading sleep expert and Director of Sleep Research at Mammoth Technologies:

❶ Create a sleeping environment – don't clutter with TVs, books or other distractions. Avoid intermittent noises and darken the room

❷ Keep cool and be comfortable – choose your mattress, pillows, duvets wisely for support, coolness and comfort

❸ Record your sleeping patterns – it may identify causes of poor sleep

Luminette

Luminette is a new, innovative light therapy device worn just like a pair of glasses. It's used to treat Seasonal Affective Disorder (SAD) and winter blues.

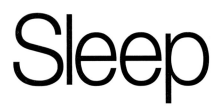

❹ Wind down routine and napping – a two hour wind down and limit naps to twenty minutes. Don't nap after 2pm.
❺ Alcohol and food – avoid alcohol and leave a period of two hours after eating a meal

SAD

Seasonal Affective Disorder (SAD) affects over two million people in the UK. Feeling stressed, depressed, lethargic, tired, irritable and having difficulty concentrating are all symptoms. It's more common in winter and seems to be down to a lack of daylight and vitamin D. Using a lightbox or a light visor such as Luminette (*www.sad-lighthire.co.uk*), may help.

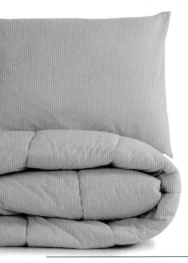

TOP TIP

"Don't head for the nearest orthopaedic bed – it may be too hard for you. Older people may have more back problems, but they also have more sensitive joints."

THE SLEEP COUNCIL, BED BUYING TIPS FOR THE OVER 50S

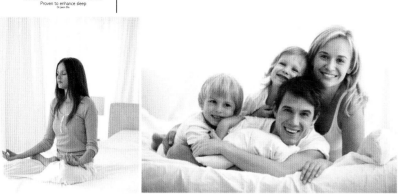

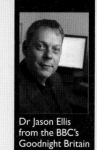

Dr Jason Ellis
from the BBC's
Goodnight Britain

SLEEP YOUR WAY TO GOOD HEALTH

What springs to mind when you think of a healthy lifestyle? Perhaps a jog around the park or tucking into a nutritious salad. But surprisingly, research has shown that the most important, and overlooked, aspect of a healthy life is the rest and recovery you get from a good night's sleep.

In fact the quality of sleep you get is not only important for your physical health but equally important to maintaining good mental health. As you sleep, your body goes into repair mode; rejuvenating body and brain.

What happens when you're asleep?

One of the key activities that occurs as you sleep is the stimulation of growth hormones, which start a process of repairing damaged cells and creating new ones. Weary muscle and brain cells are repaired and new ones created.

This is a feature that has not been lost on elite athletes or their coaches.

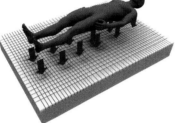

Many top sports people build in sleep recovery into their training schedule and developments in sleep science are closely followed.

Mammoth Health Mattress

One of those developments has been the Mammoth Health Mattress from Mammoth Technologies .

Using key medical-based products, the Mammoth Health Mattress has been designed to enhance sleep and create a recuperative environment for your mind and body.

Superior medical grade foam is used in preference to memory foam due to its cooling and supportive properties.

Design features such as cooling air channels and zoned support for backs, shoulders and neck have established its reputation as the ultimate health mattress.

Mammoth Technologies enlisted renowned sleep guru, and resident expert on the recent BBC series "Goodnight Britain", Dr Jason Ellis to test the innovations introduced into their mattress.

The tests were conducted at the Sleep Research Centre at Northumbria University.

The research showed categorically that the Mammoth mattress provided a more effective and enjoyable sleep. Incredibly it moved sleepers up a clinical level - turning poor sleepers into good sleepers.

This makes Mammoth mattresses the only mattresses proven to enhance sleep.

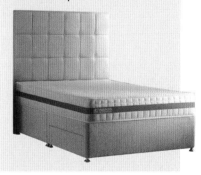

Chiropractic
Patients
Association

Partners in product design

Wake up without back pain

Hypertension

Most people don't realise they have high blood pressure until they have a check-up. It's estimated five million people in the UK have undiagnosed hypertension

High blood pressure puts you at increased risk of a heart attack or stroke, and the higher your reading, the greater your risk of health problems. Every day in the UK, 350 people have a preventable stroke or heart attack caused by high blood pressure.

Blood pressure readings are shown as two numbers. The top reading is your systolic pressure and the bottom number is your diastolic pressure. Normal blood pressure is 120/80mmHg, and at that level you have low risk of a heart attack or stroke. High blood pressure (hypertension) is usually diagnosed after a period of consistently high readings, usually 140/90mmHg.

Causes and prevention

'It is thought that being overweight, drinking too much alcohol and not doing any exercise are the main causes of high blood pressure. Sometimes however, just having a family history of high blood pressure, even without other risk factors, can increase your chances of having hypertension.

If your blood pressure is high, regular, brisk aerobic exercise is one of the most effective ways to reduce it. Recommendations are 30 minutes, five times per week. The odd stroll or gardening probably won't be enough.

Speak to your doctor before starting to exercise, and began with short sessions and build up gently. If you're overweight, losing weight will also have

a big impact on your blood pressure. If it doesn't come down with lifestyle changes or is very high, your doctor may recommend medication.

Our expert says

"We recommend everyone over 40 gets their blood pressure checked as part of a health check to assess their risk of heart and circulatory disease."
British Heart Foundation

Did you know?

Regular monitoring at home will help build up a picture of what affects your blood pressure and the effectiveness of lifestyle changes or medication. Take your readings to your doctor's appointment.*

Beet it

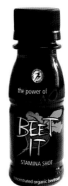

Research from the William Harvey Research Institute at Barts and the London School of Medicine (2013) suggests that drinking beetroot juice could lower blood pressure. High levels of nitrates in beetroot help to widen blood vessels and aid blood flow.
www.beet-it.com

* FOR MORE INFORMATION AND SUPPORT, GO TO BLOOD

Cholesterol

In the UK, 60% of adults have high or abnormal cholesterol, but most don't know they have a problem

Having high cholesterol increases your risk of heart disease, stroke and angina due to the build-up of atherosclerosis in the lining of the arteries. 60% of adults in the UK have raised or abnormal cholesterol levels, but there are no symptoms and most people don't realise they have a problem. Sometimes the first sign is a heart attack. According to Heart UK, the nation's cholesterol charity, around 50% of heart attacks are caused by raised cholesterol and it's the biggest medical risk factor for coronary heart disease.

What are LDL and HDL?

Cholesterol is carried around the blood by proteins called lipoproteins. LDL (low density lipoproteins) are often referred to as 'bad cholesterol' and HDL as 'good'. Knowing your ratios of HDL and LDL is important. Too much LDL is unhealthy, whereas it's good to have high levels of HDL. We need some cholesterol in our

Did you know?

"For most people, a healthy total cholesterol level is below 5 mmol/L and a healthy LDL cholesterol should be below 3 mmol/L" Heart UK, The Cholesterol Charity

blood, but too much of the wrong sort can be harmful.

Causes and prevention

'Cholesterol increases naturally as we age, but can be raised by eating a diet high in processed foods, being overweight and not being very active. Also, smoking can make cholesterol more damaging and increase your risk of heart disease.

Some people have a genetic condition known as Familial Hypercholesterolemia

GET ADVICE
Heart UK, the nation's cholesterol charity, www.heartuk.org.uk, offers lots of resources, fact sheets and support. Helpline: 08454 505 988

(FH), which can result in very high cholesterol levels and increase the risk of heart disease. It's important you receive screening and management for this condition if a close family member has very high cholesterol.

If you're over 40, you should be invited to a health check with your GP, where your cholesterol levels are checked. If not, ask for a test, or pop into your pharmacy for one.

If you're diagnosed with high cholesterol, there's a lot you can do to reduce it. Exercise, healthy eating, losing weight and not smoking or drinking alcohol can all help, particularly exercise, which can increase HDL. It isn't always easy and you'll need advice with regards to diet, so ask your GP and contact Heart UK.

Diabetes

The number of people with diabetes in the UK has increased by a staggering 36% since 2006, and there are now around three million people with the condition and a further 850,000 who are undiagnosed with Type 2 diabetes. By 2025, it's estimated that over five million people will have diabetes in the UK

Essentially, diabetes is a life-long condition affecting blood glucose levels. It can be a complex condition and, if left untreated, can lead to serious complications such as blindness, neuropathy, heart disease, stroke and kidney failure.

There are two main types of diabetes. Type 1 is where the body can't produce any insulin and it usually begins in childhood. Type 2, which is the focus here, is more common, accounting for 90% of cases, and typically develops in people over 40. It occurs when your body can't produce enough insulin or when the insulin that's produced doesn't work properly.

Did you know?

In the UK, diabetes accounts for over 10% of the NHS budget. According to Diabetes UK, in 2011 NHS spending on diabetes was £10 billion. It's also associated with 24,000 early deaths each year.

Causes

Your chances of developing Type 2 diabetes depend on a combination of genes, lifestyle and environmental factors. It's also three times more common in people from Black African and African Caribbean backgrounds, and six times more common in people from South Asian backgrounds.

Other risk factors include having a close relative with diabetes, being overweight (BMI of over 25) and having a waist measuring more than 80cm if you're a woman and 94cm for men. The main cause of Type 2 diabetes is being overweight.

Symptoms

Symptoms include increased thirst, urinating more often, extreme tiredness, unexplained weight loss, slow-healing wounds and blurred vision. Many people have Type 2 diabetes for years without knowing, as symptoms tend to develop gradually and sometimes people don't have any symptoms at all.

Jason's Story

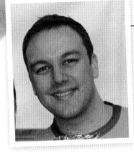

Jason McEwen was diagnosed with Type 2 diabetes in 2011 after an annual health check at work

Our expert says

"It's not a well-known fact, but there's a clear link between diabetes and gum disease," explains Richard Guyver, Dentist and Founder of the Diabetes and Dentistry Organisation. "Having inflammation in your mouth, for example from gum disease, significantly increases your risk of developing diabetes. It's therefore very important to look after your gums and mouth with regular brushing and flossing between the teeth. Bleeding from your gums is a sign of inflammation and a clear indication that you need to start taking better care of your mouth."
www.richardguyver.com

WHAT TO DO...

If you have any symptoms or are worried you're at risk of diabetes, see your GP who'll arrange a blood test. Your pharmacy can also arrange a diabetes check. See *lloydspharmacy.com.*

Find out if you're at risk by taking the Diabetes UK risk assessment (*www.diabetes.org.uk/riskscore*). Often, Type 2 diabetes is only picked up during a health check. Everyone between 40 and 74 should be invited for an NHS health check.

If you're diagnosed with diabetes, it's possible to manage your symptoms by being more active and healthy eating. Eventually, however, you may need medication. There's no cure for diabetes, so treatment should aim to keep your blood glucose levels normal.

"I had absolutely no idea that I had diabetes: I was having a bit of trouble with vertigo and my eyesight sometimes went a bit blurry, but I didn't connect this at all with diabetes. I decided that I had to completely change my lifestyle for the better. At diagnosis, I had a BMI of 34 and was obese, but since then I've lost two-and-a-half stone. I've removed all high fat and high sugar from my diet. I still spoil myself now and again, but it isn't half as frequently. I've got a personal trainer and go to the gym three or four times a week. I used training for the BUPA 10k Manchester run for Diabetes UK to focus my training schedule, and I've changed my working lifestyle to give more of a work/life balance. I have to take tablets everyday and check my blood, but I do feel much better, a lot healthier and I've got more energy. If work hadn't provided me with a private medical screening, my diabetes probably wouldn't have been picked up. If you're diagnosed with diabetes, it isn't the end of the world and there are ways of managing it. For me, managing my diabetes has actually turned around a lot of things in my life for the better."
With thanks to Diabetes UK: www.diabetes.org.uk

Osteoporosis

In the UK, there are three million people with osteoporosis and 300,000 fragility fractures a year. This skeletal disease predominantly affects people over 50

Unfortunately, osteoporosis often goes undetected until diagnosed after a fall or fracture, so the best approach is to reduce your risk by keeping your bones strong through diet and exercise.

Symptoms

If you've already broken a bone after a minor bump or fall, you may have osteoporosis, as fractures are a symptom. Other warning signs include height loss and kyphosis (curvature of the spine) due to vertebrae bones flattening or squashing.

Causes and prevention

One in two women and one in five men over the age of 50 in the UK will break a bone mainly because of bone health. The good news, say experts, is that you can address multiple lifestyle factors to help prevent osteoporosis by maintaining healthy bones.

Eat a balanced, healthy and calcium-rich diet (aim to eat 700mg of calcium every day). Get plenty of vitamin D and keep active by walking, playing tennis, dancing or running. Consider family history, as genetics play a small but significant role in bone health. You may be at risk if you've been through the menopause due to the drop in oestrogen.

> **Did you know?**
> Only 10% of our vitamin D comes from food. Opt for sunlight, but safe sun. If your skin starts to burn, your body will begin to deplete the vitamin D that it's produced, so safe sun is always best.

> **OSTEOPENIA** *means that your bone mineral density (BMD) is lower than normal, but not low enough to be classified as osteoporosis.*

"Osteoporosis is common in the UK, and women are four times more likely to develop it than men," says Professor Alan Silman, medical director at Arthritis Research UK. Men with low levels of testosterone are also at a higher risk.

Our expert says

"Be plant strong! Diet is very important in keeping bone health. It's essential to have an adequate and good calorie intake and to eat the right kinds of foods, such as those with natural phytoestrogens and foods rich in calcium and vitamin D, such as kale, spinach, beans, egg yolks and some fish. Aim to expose yourself to sunlight for 10-15 minutes a day. Avoid

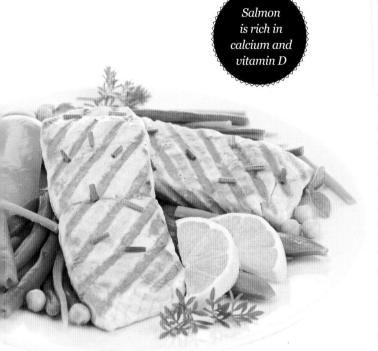

Salmon is rich in calcium and vitamin D

Fiona's Story

Fiona, 59, lives in Glasgow

"In August 2008, I sustained a hairline fracture in my ankle. When I went back to hospital the next week, a different doctor told me it wasn't a fracture, but a bad strain. That December, I was invited for a DXA scan. I nearly didn't go because I was really busy at work and, according to the Fracture Liaison Service's questionnaire, I had none of the other indicators for osteoporosis.

"Fortunately I did go, and discovered I had osteoporosis of the spine and osteopenia of the hip. The very supportive nurse gave me a booklet from the Osteoporosis Society and told me to see my GP.

"I've since taken bisphosphonates weekly, a calcium and vitamin D tablet daily, cut down on caffeine and drink more herbal teas. I've upped my fruit and veg intake and exercise more, too."

WITH THANKS TO NATIONAL OSTEOPOROSIS SOCIETY: WWW.NOS.ORG.UK; ARTHRITIS RESEARCH UK: WWW.ARTHRITISRESEARCHUK.ORG

excess alcohol and smoking. It's also a good idea to take supplements after the age of 50. Be sensible and build exercise into your routine rather than it being something you have to do. Educate yourself about fall prevention; that is, learn how to protect yourself when you fall."
Nitu Bajekal, FRCOG, Consultant Gynaecologist at Barnet and Chase Farm NHS Trust, Spire Bushey Hospital, BMI North London Hospital and the BMI Kings Oak Hospital, Hertfordshire

▲

Vitamin D
TO BOOST YOUR VITAMIN D INTAKE, TRY THE VITAMIN D ORAL SPRAY FROM BETTERYOU: BETTERYOU.UK.COM

WHAT TO DO...

If you think you're at risk talk to your GP, who'll assess your medical history, including whether you've broken any bones or lost height. You may be sent for a DXA bone scan to measure your bone density.

If you went through the menopause before the age of 45; have had a fracture as a result of a minor fall or injury; or have had corticosteroid treatments for three months or more, consider a bone scan. If diagnosed with osteoporosis, call the National Osteoporosis Society on 0845 450 0230 for an info pack and to speak with a specialist nurse.

Oral health

Gum disease affects nearly 38 million adults in the UK. It's a serious problem with significant implications for your general health. Good oral health and gum care are therefore essential

Good oral health is rather like having a fitness programme for your mouth. There are many parts and it goes much further than just preventing tooth decay or having white teeth. Eating a healthy diet low in sugar, brushing and cleaning between your teeth, using a mouth wash, and seeing your dentist and hygienist are all important considerations, as well as avoiding alcohol and smoking. Prevention is always better than cure, and there's a lot we can all do to improve our oral health.

"The two main causes of tooth loss are decay and gum disease. The better we prevent or deal with these two problems, the more chance people have of keeping their teeth for life. When the dentist, hygienist and patient work together, this can help to prevent the need for treatment and avoid the traditional pattern of fillings and extractions. Your dental team may recommend a course of treatment to get your mouth into good condition and then work out a maintenance plan to help you keep it that way." *The British Dental Health Foundation: www.dentalhealth.org*

> **" There's a lot we can all do to improve our oral health "**

Gum disease or gingivitis

Emerging research has found a strong link between oral health and the way our immune system behaves. Inflammation in the mouth – in other words, gum disease – has been found to lead to a number of chronic conditions, including diabetes, stroke and heart disease. In fact, research has shown that people with gum disease are almost three times as likely to have a heart attack than those who don't have inflammation.

"Many people have inflammation in their mouths all the time, yet don't know about it," explains Richard Guyver, dentist, author and founder of the Diabetes and Dentistry Organisation. "It's estimated that around 80% of the UK population has some form of gum disease."

Good oral health and gum care are vital and can reduce your risk of developing serious health conditions. "Brushing correctly with an electric brush (with a round, oscillating head), using fluoride toothpaste and cleaning between the teeth with floss or inter-dental brushes can all significantly improve your mouth health," explains Richard. "Bleeding gums when you brush or floss isn't normal and an indication of gum disease, so see your dentist for a check-up."

Dentistry has changed dramatically over the last 30 years, and hygienists now play a much bigger part in dental care. A hygienist will give your teeth a thorough clean, removing the build-up of plaque and show you how to get the most out of your brushing technique. Your dentist will let you know how often you should go for a check-up and how regularly you should visit the hygienist, usually every 6-12 months.

"Prevention is key when it comes to gum disease," explains Richard, "and there's a lot you can do to actively care for your mouth."

TOP TIPS

1. Don't ignore signs of gum disease, such as bleeding gums and bad breath.

2. Look after your mouth and recognise the implications on your overall health.

3. Get professional and regular intervention from a dentist and hygienist.

4. Use a toothpaste containing fluoride to help prevent decay.

5. Clean between your teeth – using floss or inter-dental brushes – twice per day and use a mouthwash in the middle of the day for a fluoride boost.
Richard Guyver: www. richardguyver.com

> *It's estimated that around 80% of the UK population has some form of gum disease*

RICHARD GUYVER GIVES PLENTY MORE ADVICE ON ORAL AND GENERAL HEALTH IN HIS BOOK.

TAKE CONTROL OF YOUR MOUTH

Ask your dentist for advice or try these:

The good news is that the early stage of gum disease is reversible if treated properly.

Colgate Pro Gum Health includes mouthwashes, toothbrushes, toothpaste, interdental brushes and floss designed to improve gum health: *www. colgate.co.uk*

UltraDEX Recalcifying & Whitening Daily Oral Rinse has been developed especially for sensitive teeth: *www. ultradex. co.uk*

TePe Interdental brushes are available in various options and sizes, including the Angle and an extra-soft version for people with inflamed dental areas: *www. tepe-interdental-brushes.co.uk*

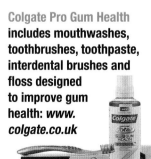

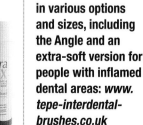

Eye health

In the UK, we value sight above all other senses, yet despite this 20 million of us fail to have our eyes checked once every two years, and 8% of adults haven't had a sight test for at least 10 years, reports the College of Optometrists

For over 50s, cataracts and age-related macular degeneration (AMD) are the leading causes of vision loss, and dry eye syndrome is the most common cause of eye irritation in over 65s. Over 600,000 people in the UK have AMD, and 96% of people over 60 need some form of vision correction, according to research from The Eyecare Trust.

Contact lens care

Make sure your hands are clean before touching your lenses. Avoid showering, sleeping or swimming with them in, as you risk developing a serious eye infection. Be strict about cleaning your contacts, using only the solution recommended by your practitioner.

Our expert says

"People need to understand what's happening to their sight, so they should read up and become informed, and have a regular eye check. It's also vital to wear a quality pair of sunglasses, because it's light that tends to damage the structures in the eye. Also, for many people, the surface of their eyes starts drying with age. A diet adequate in omega 3 and 6 helps in the production of the type of moisture needed." *Milind Pande, Medical Director and Consultant Ophthalmic Surgeon at Vision Surgery and Research Centre*

TOP TIPS

1 It's worth wearing good-quality sunglasses in the sun or in high-glare areas, as exposure to UV rays may contribute to eye problems such as cataracts and AMD

2 The nutrients in omega-3 fatty acids, in zinc and in vitamins C and E may also help to prevent age-related vision issues – so try on green, leafy veg

3 Read up on family history: there are genetic links to AMD as well as to glaucoma and squint

4 Wear protective eye wear when playing sports or for DIY work; 20,000 eye accidents occur every year due to DIY

5 Screen fatigue includes sore, itchy or tired eyes; headaches; impaired colour perception and temporary blurred vision. Computer breaks are key.

WHAT TO DO...

Sight tests are vital, so get your eyes tested regularly. Not only can optometrists identify eye conditions such as glaucoma before they cause irreversible sight loss, they can also reveal other serious medical conditions such as hypertension, high cholesterol, diabetes and the risk of stroke.

Sexual health

There are many proven health benefits of being sexually active, including improved immunity, lowered blood pressure, reduced stress and increased life expectancy. Lots of reasons to stay sexually active!

Gets better with age

Many people say their sex life actually gets better with age, thanks to less pressure, feeling more confident and relaxed, and having more time. Physically, sex might not be quite the same as it was in your youth, but it can be more enjoyable than ever, strengthening your relationship with your partner.

But things can change as you get older, and sex can become difficult due to factors such as menopause or ill health. Vaginal dryness after the menopause is experienced by around three million women in the UK, making intercourse

SEEKING SUPPORT
If you're worried about your health and having sex, or are experiencing problems, it's important to speak to your GP

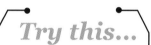

Try this...
Over-the-counter gel Balance Activ

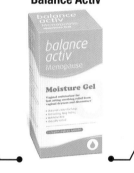

painful or uncomfortable. Your GP may prescribe HRT, or try using an over-the-counter gel or pessary such as Balance Activ, *www.balanceactiv.com.*

Erection problems can affect a man at any age, although it does become more common as you get older, especially over 65. Around 40% of men aged 60-69 are thought to have erectile dysfunction. But erection problems aren't a natural process of ageing and there may be an underlying medical condition requiring

treatment. See your GP if you're having problems.

Our expert says

"Many couples find it frustrating that their bodies aren't working in the same way as they used to. Sexual pleasure tends to change, but it doesn't mean you can't still enjoy being sexual together. Many couples find their sex life improves as changes in their health helps them be more creative." *Paula Hall, Sexual Psychotherapist and author of 'Improving Your Relationship for Dummies'*

Safe sex

The incidence of sexually transmitted diseases has increased dramatically in people aged 45-64 over the last decade. In men aged 45-64, chlamydia increased by 264% between 2003-2011. It's thought this is due to an increase in older single people enjoying new sexual freedom. It's important to talk to a new partner about using condoms.

Cystitis

A urine infection in the bladder is common in women, but less so among men. One in five women will suffer from recurrent cystitis

Cystitis is an inflammation of the bladder – sometimes referred to as a urinary tract infection, or UTI – and it can be very painful. Half of all women will have had a bout of it at least once in their lifetime, and about one in five will have recurrent cystitis. It's more common if you're post-menopausal due to changes in hormonal levels.

Cystitis is less common among men, but more serious, as it could indicate something more sinister such as a bladder or prostate problem, or an obstruction of the urinary tract.

Symptoms

A burning sensation when urinating, or needing to wee more often and with urgency but only passing small amounts. Watch out for dark-coloured, cloudy or strong-smelling urine. You may feel unwell, have a fever or have pain in your lower belly. While symptoms can be obvious, cystitis doesn't always present typically, particularly in older women who may just feel off colour.

What about cranberry juice? There's little evidence about cranberry juice in the treatment of cystitis, but taking high-strength tablets may have a role in prevention.

Expert view

"Don't ignore recurrent cystitis (more than three episodes in a year), as there may be an underlying condition such as a kidney stone that needs treatment. It's important to notify your doctor if you notice any visible blood in your urine, as this can sometimes be a sign of something more serious. Cystitis is rare in men and warrants further tests, as it may be an indication of an underlying prostate problem."
Rashmi Singh, Consultant Urological Surgeon, St Anthony's Hospital

WHAT TO DO...

Very mild cases can be treated with cystitis relief sachets, which can be bought over the counter, and by drinking lots of water, but it may not clear the infection. "If symptoms persist or you have more serious symptoms, such as blood in your urine, it's essential to go and see your GP. Normally, urinary tract infections need to be treated with antibiotics," advises GP Dr Sarah Jarvis.

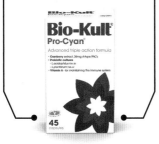

Pelvic floor

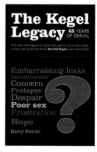

It's estimated that around 42% of women in the UK suffer from pelvic floor problems. Don't ignore them

Think of your pelvic floor as a hammock that runs from your pubic bone at the front to the base of your spine at the back. Referred to as the pubococcygeus (PC), it's responsible for bowel and bladder control in both men and women, and essentially holds all your pelvic organs in place in the pelvis.

The onset of menopause can cause your pelvic floor muscles to weaken further as levels of oestrogen drop. A weak pelvic floor can be hugely distressing, leading to urine incontinence, vaginal prolapse, bowel incontinence and sexual problems, including erectile dysfunction in men, too.

Our expert says

"Many women are aware of the need for pelvic floor exercises, but few carry them out regularly and effectively," explains Barry Fowler, author of *The Kegel Legacy, www.thekegellegacy.com*. "The techniques recommended are

Try this...

There are many products to help strengthen your pelvic floor. Ask your GP or physiotherapist which is most suitable for you. The PelvicToner is the only one available on prescription: *www. pelvictoner.co.uk* Some women may find an electronic device such as the Kegel 8Ultra works for them: www.kegel8.co.uk

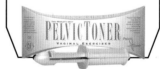

often not rigorous enough and fall short of the clinically proven exercises recommended by Arnold Kegel many years ago. Using an exercise device that helps you correctly identify the muscles to squeeze and ideally provides some sort

of resistance is important. There needs to be an element of effort: it's like weight training without weights."

Don't ignore it!

The message, however, is clear; you shouldn't ignore problems with your pelvic floor. It will continue to get worse unless you seek treatment. It's estimated that it can take women up to ten years before they seek help. Don't be one of them. Help is available and you shouldn't suffer in silence.

There's a lot you can do yourself with the correct exercises and identification of the right muscles. Take control of the problem: see your GP for advice, referral to a specialist or ask to see a physiotherapist who specialises in women's health.

BARRY FOWLER OFFERS MORE ADVICE IN HIS BOOK.

Osteoarthritis

Osteoarthritis is the most common form of arthritis in the UK. More than one million people consult their GP about the condition every year

Mainly affecting people over the age of 45, it's not known exactly how many people suffer from osteoarthritis (OA), but data gathered by Arthritis Research UK suggests that more than six million people in the UK have OA in one or both knees and around 8.5 million people have X-ray evidence of OA in the spine.

It can affect any joint in the body, but most commonly is found in the spine, and typically occurs in the knees, hips and small joints of the hands and big toe. There are around 140,000 knee and hip replacements performed annually due to the condition.

Symptoms

Osteoarthritis occurs when there's a loss of cartilage at the end of the joint and the main symptom is pain. The symptoms vary from person to person and may even be different between affected joints. The main characteristics are inflammation of the tissues in and around the joints, damage to the cartilage and bony growths that develop around the edges of the joints. Symptoms are generally pain, stiffness and difficulty performing certain activities.

Our expert says

"It's a myth that exercise is bad for people with arthritis. Numerous studies have shown that moderate exercise can be beneficial for some people with arthritic joints. Gentle aerobic exercise such as brisk walking, cycling or rowing may help reduce the chronic low-grade inflammation associated with 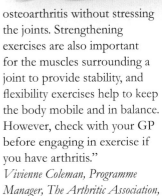 osteoarthritis without stressing the joints. Strengthening exercises are also important for the muscles surrounding a joint to provide stability, and flexibility exercises help to keep the body mobile and in balance. However, check with your GP before engaging in exercise if you have arthritis."
Vivienne Coleman, Programme Manager, The Arthritic Association, www.arthriticassociation.org.uk

Did you know?

Research from the University of East Anglia has discovered that eating broccoli could slow or prevent the progress of the most common form of arthritis. Sulforaphane, found in broccoli, could slow the destruction of cartilage, which is associated with osteoarthritis: www.*arthritisresearchuk.org*

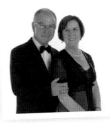

Jim's Story

Jim, aged 69 from Gloucestershire, took up walking and lost four stone

"Back in 2008, I was square and squat and I knew I was too heavy for my knees. The pain from my arthritis never stopped me walking, but it was constant. I was 65, coming into official retirement, but fat and unfit. My brother had also just been diagnosed with liver cancer and it was a huge shock. I knew things had to change. I started to attend my local Slimming World group and I found it worked well for me.

"At the same time, I started to walk three miles a day at 5am. Gradually, I lost weight and got fitter. I'm now a trim 12.5 stone and walk up to eight miles a day. Losing weight and exercising worked well together – the one encouraged the other. As I lost weight, the pain in my knee gradually reduced, and it's practically gone now. "I used to have a problem walking, especially downhill, but now I'm pain-free. I'm also fitter, have more energy and my blood pressure is back to normal."

WITH THANKS TO ARTHRITIS RESEARCH UK

WHAT TO DO...

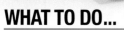

Getting medical help is important. Not all aches and pains are due to OA and could be down to other musculoskeletal conditions. Some may be more serious than others, so always visit your GP, who may refer you to a rheumatologist for further tests and investigations. Treatment options will depend on your diagnosis, and you may be referred to a surgeon, neurologist, physiotherapist or other specialist. There are many types of medications, drugs and complementary therapies to treat arthritis, and you need to discuss all options with your GP. There's also a lot of conflicting advice on the internet and in the media about diet and supplements, so it's important to speak to your GP about this, too

There is strong evidence that being a healthy weight, exercising regularly and eating a balanced, mediterranean-style diet helps: *www.arthriticassociation.org.uk*

Bowel health

None of us like to talk about our bowels, but a lack of awareness could mean your digestive system is less than optimum, potentially affecting your quality of life

I t's estimated that a third of the UK population regularly suffer from a digestive-related problem. Bloating, constipation, diarrhoea, pain, wind, nausea and sickness are common and often made worse with stress. Eating a healthy, balanced diet, drinking enough water and limiting alcohol all help to avoid bowel problems, as well as maintaining a healthy weight, exercising regularly and taking a probiotic supplement.

Constipation
A study published in 2013 by The International Longevity Centre UK, *www.ilcuk.org.uk*, reported that 80% of people living in care homes and one in five adults over 65 in the community are affected by constipation. According to the report, constipation is a serious condition that's widely under-estimated,

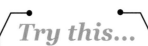
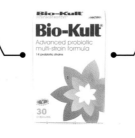
under-treated and overlooked. If left untreated, it can lead to serious medical problems.

What about IBS?
Irritable Bowel Syndrome, or IBS, is the name doctors give to a collection of otherwise unexplained symptoms affecting the colon or large bowel. Symptoms are widely varied and include abdominal pain and spasms, diarrhoea, constipation and/or an erratic bowel habit, bloating or swelling of the stomach and excessive wind. IBS affects around 35% of the population and is linked with stress.

Diverticular disease
Diverticular disease is where small grape-sized pouches protrude out of the colon and is common in older people. They usually don't cause a problem, but can get inflamed, leading to diverticulitis. Symptoms include pain (usually on the left side), change in bowel habit or blood in your bowel motion. See your GP if you have any symptoms.

Seek help
Although you may feel embarrassed talking to your GP about your bowels, it's essential to get a medical diagnosis to rule out more serious disorders. Find out more at *www.bladderandbowelfoundation.org* or call the helpline on 0845 345 0165.

An introduction to
cancer

The chances are that you know someone who's been affected by cancer, possibly a close relative, colleague or perhaps even yourself. It's the nation's biggest fear and understandably so, as it's estimated one in three people will develop some form of cancer during their lifetime

Cancer rates have risen dramatically since the mid-1970s, and today around 890 people are diagnosed with cancer every day in the UK.

There are more than 200 types of cancer, each with different symptoms, causes and treatments. Some cancers are more prevalent than others, and there has been the biggest increase in cancers linked to lifestyle, such as kidney, liver, skin, oral and uterine cancers. Over the next few pages, we'll talk about some of the most common cancers that affect people over the age of 50 and what you need to watch out for.

Your risk of developing cancer depends on many variables, including your age, gender, lifestyle, genetics and family history. According to the World Cancer Research Fund, around 38% of the most common cancers in the UK could be prevented through improved diet, physical activity and weight management. A study by Cancer Research UK, however,

showed that a third of people questioned believed their chance of getting cancer was down to fate and they couldn't do anything about it.

There is, in fact, a lot we can

> *" Around 38% of the most common cancers in the UK could be prevented through improved diet, physical activity and weight management "*

do to try and avoid getting cancer in the first place. If you were offered a simple way to lower your risk of developing cancer, you'd

take it. Making healthier lifestyle choices, such as not smoking, keeping a healthy weight, improved diet, physical activity and weight management are all things you can do to reduce your risk. Cancer can be preventable and you have the power to influence it.

Even though the number of people diagnosed with cancer is rising, the good news is that the survival rate has doubled in the last 40 years due to increased awareness, ongoing research, better detection and medical treatment.

Being aware of symptoms is vital, as many cancers can be successfully treated if caught early. It would be easy to flick over the following pages or ignore them altogether; the subject of cancer doesn't make for light entertainment after all. But reading about the symptoms of cancer and becoming more aware is one of the most important things you can do and may well end up saving your life.

Bowel cancer

Bowel cancer is the third most common cancer in the UK, affecting 40,000 people a year. Both men and women are equally at risk, and 95% of patients diagnosed with bowel cancer are over the age of 55

 lso referred to as colorectal cancer (as the majority of cancers are found in the colon or rectum), it's one of the most treatable cancers if caught quickly, and there's a high survival rate in patients diagnosed at an early stage.

Sadly, though, bowel cancer is still responsible for 16,000 deaths a year, making it the second biggest cancer killer in the UK.

Screening

Bowel cancer screening is widely available to people aged between 60 and 69 in the UK (*www.cancerscreening.nhs.uk/bowel*). The home testing kit looks for hidden blood in your stool (Faecal Occult Blood), which can detect the early stages of cancer before you notice any symptoms. It's important you

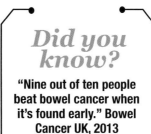

Did you know?

"Nine out of ten people beat bowel cancer when it's found early." Bowel Cancer UK, 2013

take up this offer of screening and send back the completed testing kit. If you're over the age of 70, you can request a kit by calling 0800 707 6060. If blood is found in your sample, you'll be asked to see your GP for further testing. If you're under the age of 60, you won't be sent a kit automatically, but you can purchase your own from *www.medichecks.com*.

Symptoms

The main signs and symptoms of bowel cancer include blood in your stool, bleeding from your bottom and repeated loose bowel movements, especially if lasting longer than three weeks. Other symptoms include a pain or lump in your stomach, weight loss for no obvious reason and feeling more tired than usual.

Some of these symptoms could be mistaken for other conditions, such as haemorrhoids or IBS, which is why seeing your doctor straightaway is so important. None of us want to talk about our bowels and many people understandably find it embarrassing, but awareness of the symptoms of cancer and making an appointment to see your doctor if you're worried could actually end up saving your life.

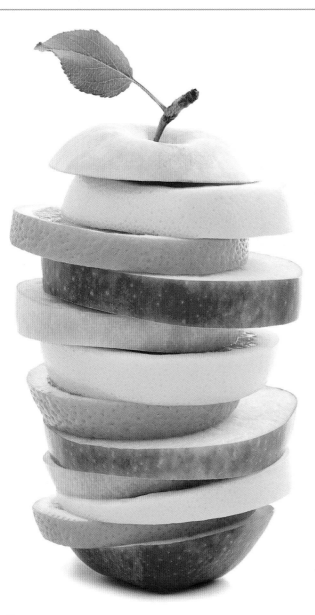

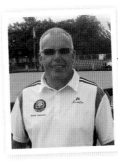

Sandy's story

Sandy, 62, from Perth in Scotland was diagnosed with bowel cancer in May 2003

"After I received the screening test in the post, I had to be persuaded by my wife to do it. I almost sent it back without doing it at all! But it's a decision that I now know saved my life. If I'd put off taking the test, my situation would have been very serious and, if I'd left it any longer, I may not have been here today to spend time with my grandchildren. Taking the test was crucial to my survival.

"I was so shocked. I never thought cancer would happen to me, I was a regular runner, non-smoker and prided myself on always being fit and well. Treatment began straightaway. I underwent surgery and a course of chemotherapy.

"So many fantastic things have happened since my diagnosis. I've become a grandfather and my daughter has married. I was very lucky to have my condition diagnosed early and I'm keen to raise awareness about getting signs and symptoms checked out."

WITH THANKS TO CANCER RESEARCH UK: FREEPHONE 0808 800 4040; WWW.CANCERRESEARCHUK.ORG

Our expert says

"Many cases of bowel cancer are linked to lifestyle, and there are lots of things you can do to help lower the risk of the disease. Keeping to a healthy weight, eating plenty of fibre, fruit and veg, limiting red and processed meat and alcohol, staying physically active and not smoking can all help towards reducing the risk. A healthy lifestyle isn't a guarantee against cancer, but it helps stack the odds in your favour."
Adeyinka Ebo, Senior Health Information Officer, Cancer Research UK

WHAT TO DO...

Whether you're invited in after screening or have noticed symptoms, your doctor will examine you and may arrange further tests or referral to a specialist consultant. It's important to make a list of your symptoms and to try not to feel embarrassed or awkward.

Ovarian
cancer

Ovarian cancer predominantly affects older women, with 80% of cases occurring over the age of 50, particularly in those who have reached the menopause

Unfortunately, many women are only diagnosed at an advanced stage, as the symptoms tend to be quite vague and are easily missed, confused for other conditions such as diverticulitis, IBS or a urine infection. While ovarian cancer is relatively uncommon, the disease still accounts for 4,400 deaths each year, more than all the other gynaecological cancers put together. Awareness of symptoms is therefore vitally important.

Symptoms

Watch out for lower abdominal pain, persistent bloating and swelling of the abdomen. There may also be bowel or urinary changes – needing to urinate more often – reduced appetite, early satiety and weight loss or gain. Be alert to the symptoms of ovarian cancer and never make the assumption that any changes are due to age or diet.

Causes and prevention

You might be more at risk of ovarian cancer if you started menstruating at a young age or have a late menopause. Women who haven't had children are also at greater risk, as well as those who suffer from other gynaecological conditions such as endometriosis, ovarian cysts or infertility. Having a body mass index (BMI) above 30 or taking HRT are also thought to slightly increase your risk of developing the disease.

Our expert says

"Many women with very early ovarian cancer have no symptoms at all and

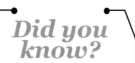

Did you know?

"If your symptoms suggest there's a chance that you could have ovarian cancer, your GP should offer you a blood test, to measure the levels of a protein called CA125 in your blood. If your CA125 is increased to a level that may suggest ovarian cancer, your GP should arrange for you to have an ultrasound of your abdomen and pelvis." NICE clinical guidelines, 2011

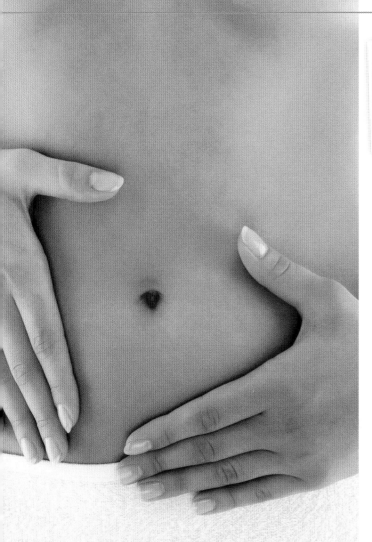

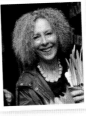

Lou's story

Lou Pescod, 62, lives in Somerset with her husband

"Bloating was the main symptom for me and what really made me go to my GP. It became so awful that I pointed it out to my sister and she urged me to see a doctor. I went to my GP, but she dismissed my symptoms as being a urinary infection. The symptoms didn't go, so I went back and was referred for a scan.

"I had surgery in December 2008 to have what I thought was a cyst removed. I was diagnosed with Clear Cell Carcinoma of the right ovary. I was very lucky the tumour had been self-contained within the ovary and that it had all been removed. My oncologist opted for the belt and braces approach, and I had three months of chemotherapy, my treatment was over by 2010.

"If you're worried or have persistent bloating, go straight to the doctor. Don't put it down to age or diet; it could be more serious. I lead a very active life and work almost full time. My husband and I love to go to the theatre or the cinema, and I'm always in London to see my children."

WITH THANKS TO OVARIAN CANCER ACTION: WWW.OVARIAN.ORG.UK

don't even know they have the disease. However, the outcome can be very positive if caught early. The five-year survival rate in patients with early-stage cancer is almost 90%."

Stephen Attard-Montalto, Consultant Gynaecologist, Nuffield Hospital, Tunbridge Wells, Kent

WHAT TO DO...

It's important to see your GP, especially if you experience a number of symptoms, in particular bloating of your stomach. Remember to mention any family history of breast or ovarian cancer, especially in a close relative such as a mother or sister. If your symptoms don't go away or get worse, go back to your GP and ask to be re-examined and for a second opinion.

If you need further investigations, you'll be referred to a gynaecologist, where under NHS guidelines you should be seen within two weeks. If you ask to be referred privately to see a consultant, you're usually seen more quickly.

Breast cancer

*Every year, nearly 55,000 people are diagnosed with breast cancer.
It's now the most common cancer in the UK*

Increased awareness and improved detection and treatments mean that survival rates from breast cancer are improving significantly, with more than eight out ten people surviving beyond five years.

Causes and prevention

Our risk of developing breast cancer increases as we get older. 80% of cases are found in women over the age of 50, so it's much more common in women who've gone through the menopause. It's rare in younger women, although still around 10,000 are diagnosed each year. Family history is an important factor for some, but this only accounts for less than 10% of breast cancer cases overall. Lifestyle choices, environmental factors and genetics all have a part to play in this complex disease, there are many factors we can't control. "There's also good evidence that women can reduce the risk of developing breast cancer by keeping a healthy weight, drinking less alcohol and being physically active," says Adeyinka Ebo, Cancer Research UK

Did you know?

Although rare, breast cancer also affects men - around 400 cases each year. Symptoms in men include a lump around the nipple or other area of the breast tissue, nipple discharge, tender nipple, swelling or ulceration of the breast or swelling under the arm. Don't be embarrassed. See your GP if you're worried or have any symptoms.

Symptoms

Changes to look out for include any sort of lump or thickening of the breast tissue, a change in size or shape of your breast, changes in skin texture such as dimpling or puckering of the skin, a change in the shape of your nipple or it becoming inverted, discharge from the nipple, a rash on the nipple or surrounding area, constant pain the breast or armpit, or any sort of swelling or lump in your armpit. Many of these symptoms won't necessarily mean you have cancer, but they do need to be checked out by your GP.

Screening

In the UK, the NHS breast cancer screening programme is available to all women between 50 and 70. You'll receive a letter every three years inviting you to have a mammogram. If anything

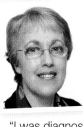

Berenice's Story

Berenice Cowan, 58, lives in Cheshire

"I was diagnosed with breast cancer in 2009 when I was 54 years old. I had pain in my armpit and then found a lump in my breast. The news that it was breast cancer was devastating. I had six months of treatment, starting with chemotherapy to reduce the size of the tumour and then a mastectomy followed by radiotherapy. I've taken Tamoxifen and I'm now on Letrozole.

"I saw a friend's scar before I had my surgery and was also shown what a prosthesis looked like so I felt really prepared. After my mastectomy, I decided against reconstruction and also chose to have a second mastectomy, and I don't feel any less feminine.

"I've been through ups and downs with this, but I'm still me! I've been supported by family and friends. I model at Breast Cancer Care Lingerie Evenings, a real confidence booster, and it's amazing to support other women in a similar situation."

IF YOU HAVE ANY QUESTIONS, CALL BREAST CANCER CARE'S FREE HELPLINE 0808 800 6000 OR FIND OUT MORE AT WWW.BREASTCANCERCARE.ORG.UK.

unusual is found, you'll be asked to go back for further tests. NICE guidelines recommend that women in their 40s who have a significantly higher risk of breast cancer should have annual mammograms.

Our expert says

"There's no right or wrong way to check your breasts – the most important thing to do is look at and feel your breasts regularly. Most changes won't turn out to be breast cancer, but don't be scared of talking to your doctor or delay going for a check-up, as the sooner the diagnosis, the more effective treatment may be."
Emma Pennery, Clinical Director at Breast Cancer Care

WHAT TO DO...

See your doctor straight away if you notice anything different in your breasts. Nine out of ten are benign (not cancer), but it's vital to see your GP to rule it out. According to NICE guidelines in the UK, if your symptoms suggest breast cancer you should get an appointment with a specialist within two weeks. There are many conditions that are benign, so your GP may adopt a wait and see approach.

Lung cancer

Lung cancer is the most common cancer in the world, with around 40,000 people diagnosed each year in the UK

Over 80% of people diagnosed with lung cancer are over the age of 60 and it's more common in men than in women. Sadly, it's the biggest killer in the UK, accounting for 35,000 deaths every year – that's more than breast, prostate, bladder cancer and leukaemia put together.

There are many different types of lung cancer, however, some of which grow relatively slowly and some that develop and spread more rapidly. It's a distressing and complex disease, and can be hard to diagnose in its early stages. It's also one of the most difficult cancers to treat and is often found when the disease is quite far advanced. However, when caught early, treatment is often very effective and many patients can be cured by surgery or other treatments.

Causes

Lung cancer is closely linked to a history of cigarette smoking, which causes nearly 86% of cases. A further 3% are caused by exposure to smoke in non-smokers. You're more likely to get lung cancer if you smoke heavily or have been smoking a long time.

There are however, an increasing number of cases in people who've never smoked, especially in women.

Other cases of lung cancer

> 66 *Lung cancer accounts for 35,000 deaths a year in the UK* 99

are linked to exposure to certain chemicals and gases, air pollution, previous lung disease, previous cancer treatment and family history.

Symptoms

Symptoms include a persistent cough or change in a long-standing cough, becoming breathless and wheezy, coughing up blood-stained phlegm, chest or shoulder pain, weight loss, chest infections, a hoarse voice, a dull ache or sharp pain when you take a deep breath, and feeling tired and lethargic.

Our expert says

"While stopping smoking is the most important thing you can do to reduce your risk of developing lung cancer, there's also evidence to suggest that eating a diet rich in antioxidants (found in foods such as fruit and fresh vegetables) can reduce your risk of the disease. Conversely, a diet too heavy in saturated fats, such as meat and dairy products, seems to increase your risk of lung cancer. Regular exercise and keeping your weight down have also been shown to reduce the risk."

Dr Mick Peake, Consultant in respiratory medicine, Glenfield Hospital, Leicester, and Chair of the Clinical Reference Group of the UK Lung Cancer Coalition

Kathy's Story

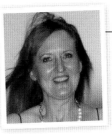

Kathy, 58, from Lincolnshire was diagnosed with a rare form of lung cancer in 2007

"I'd been suffering with lots of coughs and colds for months and I was diagnosed with asthma, which was treated with an inhaler. During 2007, I was suffering from terrible pain in my side, which caused difficulty in breathing. The doctor diagnosed pleurisy and prescribed antibiotics. After about a week, I became quite ill and was taken to hospital, where I was diagnosed with pneumonia. I was X-rayed and it was then that something was noticed on my right lung. A scan and biopsy revealed I had an adenoid cystic carcinoma, a rare form of lung cancer that I'd probably had for about four years.

"I was devastated. After never smoking and having what I thought was a healthy lifestyle, how could I have lung cancer? Two weeks later, I found myself in hospital having a lung removed. I then underwent five weeks of intensive radiotherapy. The side effects were debilitating and I found it difficult to eat or drink. I felt pretty awful. But, on 9 December, I finished my radiotherapy and began to recover with the help of my wonderful daughters, family and friends.

"It's six years since my surgery and radiotherapy, and I feel really good. I have six-monthly check-ups with my oncologist. I love to walk and dance and, while it's not always easy with one lung, I live life to the full and I'm so happy to be alive."

Did you know?

As soon as you stop smoking, your risk goes down, no matter how old you are. After ten years, your risk of lung cancer falls to around half that of a smoker. For more information on quitting, go to *www.ash.org.uk.*

WHAT TO DO...

Although many symptoms of lung cancer can be caused by other conditions, it's vital to see your GP, especially if you've had the symptoms for over three weeks. Your GP will arrange a chest X-ray, and if cancer is suspected you'll be referred to a consultant for tests, advice and treatment. You should be seen within two weeks.

WITH THANKS TO ROY CASTLE LUNG CANCER FOUNDATION: WWW.ROYCASTLE.ORG; HELPLINE 0333 323 7200

Prostate cancer

It's estimated that about one in eight men will get prostate cancer at some point in their lives, and it's now the most common male cancer in the UK. On average, over 40,000 men are diagnosed every year

Many cases of prostate cancer develop very slowly and may never cause symptoms or require treatment in a man's lifetime. Other forms are more aggressive and will need treatment to prevent the cancer spreading, which is why men, especially those with a family history of the disease, should be vigilant to the possible symptoms and seek advice from their GP.

Causes and prevention

Prostate cancer generally affects men over the age of 50 and is rare in younger men. Around 80% of men over the age of 80 will have some cancer cells in their prostate, although these cells can grow very slowly and may never need treatment.

Having a family history of

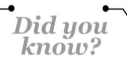

Did you know?

Men who have relatives with breast cancer may also have a higher risk of prostate cancer, particularly if the family members were diagnosed under the age of 60

cancer seems to be the biggest risk factor. Generally speaking, if you had a father or brother with prostate cancer, you're two-and-a-half times more likely to get it yourself. A study from the University of California has also shown that men who've had colon cancer may be more at risk, and that men who have a first-degree relative who's had bladder cancer are also at increased risk.

The disease is also more common in African-Caribbean men than white or Asian men. African-Caribbean men are three times more likely to get prostate cancer than white men of the same age in the UK. It's not clear why, but it seems to be due to a mixture of inherited genes and environmental factors.

Symptoms

Some men don't have any symptoms, but things to look out for include urinary frequency, getting up at night to pass water, urinary urgency and a poor stream. Other indications may include difficulty starting to pass urine, a feeling that your bladder hasn't completely emptied and dribbling urine.

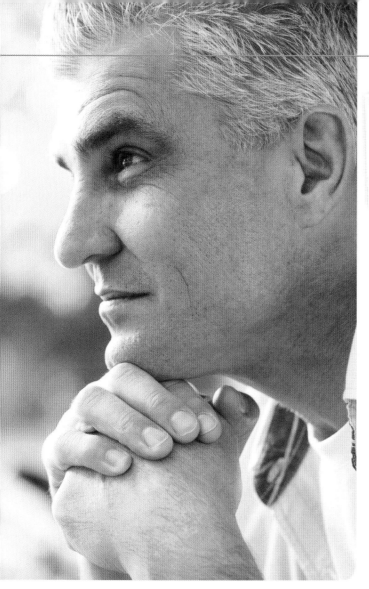

Simon's Story

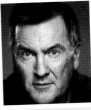

Simon D'Arcy lives in **Bordon, Hampshire, with his wife**

"I was 58 years old and didn't have any symptoms, so had never given it a second thought and didn't think I'd be at risk of prostate cancer. My wife suggested I should get a PSA blood test at my local surgery as she'd read about the risk of prostate cancer being higher in older men and thought it would be a good idea. The result came back with a raised PSA level, which triggered three more tests and a biopsy, which finally confirmed I had prostate cancer. I was diagnosed on Valentine's Day in 2009. I opted for surgery and haven't required any more treatment.

"I was a fit and active non-smoker; I was stunned. I couldn't understand why it was me. I always thought if I had prostate cancer, I'd know about it. I couldn't have been more wrong. Asking my GP for a PSA test was easily the best decision I ever made."

WITH THANKS TO PROSTATE CANCER UK: WWW.PROSTATECANCERUK.ORG; HELPLINE 0800 074 8383

Our expert says

"Deciding on the best treatment for prostate cancer isn't always straightforward, and a diagnosis of the disease doesn't always mean that it will cause problems or be life threatening. Not all men who are diagnosed with early disease will need treatment. One of the concerns in diagnosing early prostate cancer is the potential for over-treatment, causing an adverse effect on the quality of life, particularly bladder, bowel and sexual side effects. However, for those who have more advance-staged cancer, newer treatments including surgery and radiotherapy are generally highly successful."

Andrew Adamson, Consultant Urological Surgeon at The Nuffield Hospital, Wessex Chandlers Ford, Hampshire

WHAT TO DO...

Don't ignore any symptoms and make an appointment with your GP, especially if you have a family history of prostate cancer. One of the tests used to look for changes to the prostate, include the PSA which measures the total Prostate Specific Antigen (PSA) in your blood. A raised level may indicate you have a problem with your prostate, but not necessarily cancer. It can indicate further tests are needed such as a rectal examination, biopsy of the prostate gland, MRI, CT or bone scans.

Other
cancers

It is thought that up to 38% of all cancers could be prevented by changes to lifestyle, and there are many things we can do to reduce our risk of the disease

There are over 200 types of cancer. The most common in the UK today are bowel, breast, prostate, lung and ovarian, but many others are becoming more prevalent due to lifestyle choices.

Skin cancer

Malignant melanoma skin cancer is the fifth most common cancer in the UK, affecting around 13,000 people every year. Skin cancer is more common in older people, but a third of cases are found in people under the age of 55. Over the last 30 years, the incidence of malignant melanoma has risen faster than any other cancer, which experts think is linked to excessive sun exposure.

The most common sites to develop malignant melanoma are on the chest and back for men, and on the leg for women.

Symptoms

Symptoms of melanoma are a new mole, skin change or a mole that's getting bigger or changing shape and/or colour; or a mole that's itchy or sore, bleeding or looking crusty or inflamed. You should always

> ❝ *Be aware of your moles, how they look and be observant for any changes* ❞

see your doctor as soon as possible, as pre-cancerous moles are easy to treat and remove. Leaving them means the cancer could spread and be more difficult to treat. Be aware of your moles, how they look and be observant for any changes.

Oral cancer

There are a number of cancers that develop in the mouth, oral cavity, lips, tongue and throat, and they're grouped together as oral cancer. Around 6,500 people were diagnosed with some type of oral cancer in 2010, and this figure is rising steadily. Oral cancers are linked closely to smoking, alcohol consumption and infection with the HPV virus. More than half the cases in the UK may be linked to insufficient fruit and vegetable intake. Your dentist is often the first person to spot signs of oral cancer, so regular check-ups are important.

Symptoms

Ongoing pain or discomfort in the mouth is a common symptom of mouth cancer and should be reported to your doctor or dentist. A sore area (ulcer) that doesn't heal or an abnormal-looking patch in the

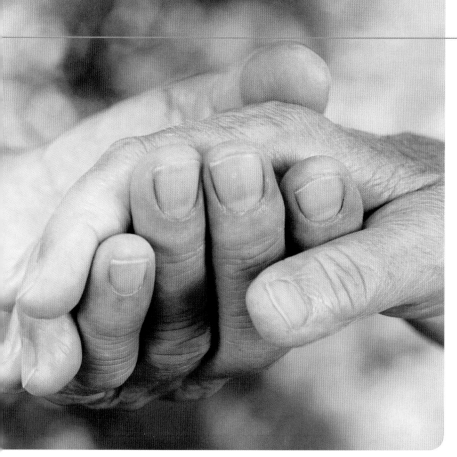

Womb cancer

Around 8,300 women are diagnosed with womb cancer in the UK each year. It's the fourth most common cancer in women in the UK and occurs mostly in women between 60 and 79. It isn't known what exactly causes it, but one of the biggest risk factors is being overweight. Women who are obese are two to three times more likely to develop the disease. This is because fat cells are linked to a higher level of oestrogen, which can cause the lining of the womb to thicken, therefore increasing the risk of it becoming cancerous. A rare genetic condition known as HNPCC is associated with an increased risk of both womb and bowel cancer. If you have close relatives with bowel and womb cancer, speak to your GP about genetic screening.

Symptoms

The most common symptom is bleeding, especially in women who've gone through the menopause. Over 90% of cases are picked up because of abnormal vaginal bleeding. Other symptoms include pain in the lower abdomen, discomfort during intercourse, loss of appetite, weight loss, tiredness, constipation or passing urine more often.

For more information on all cancers, go to *www.cancerresearch.uk.org*.

mouth could be sign of cancer or pre-cancerous changes. Any sort of lump or swelling, difficult swallowing or speaking, weight loss or bad breath could all be symptoms, so see your GP straightaway.

Liver cancer

Cancer of the liver is rare, but on the increase, and there are around 4,200 cases of primary liver cancer in the UK a year. It's more common in men than women, and around 90% of cases are diagnosed in people over 55. Damage to the liver caused by cirrhosis (scarring) increases your risk of liver cancer. Long-term heavy drinking is one of the biggest risk factors in developing liver cancer, as well as smoking, being overweight and previous infection with hepatitis B or C.

Symptoms

Symptoms include weight loss, loss of appetite, feeling sick, bloating or pain in the stomach. Yellow skin, dark urine and pale faeces are also signs. Many of the symptoms are relatively vague, making it difficult to diagnose. See your doctor if you have any of the symptoms. If you're at a higher risk, you may be offered an ultrasound every six months to check for growths in your liver.

Getting the best from
YOUR GP

You should never put off seeing your doctor if you're concerned about any aspect of your health

Your GP is your first port of call if you're unwell or need medical advice. You should be able to see your doctor whenever you need to; whether you're feeling ill, anxious, depressed or need advice or treatment for a medical condition, or simply have concerns about your risk of developing a problem.

But your GP is under growing pressure and their workloads are rising. According to a recent report, the average GP consultation in the UK lasts eight to ten minutes, leading both doctors and patients to feel under pressure and rushed.

It's also estimated that many common conditions, such as coughs, colds, back pain and headaches, many of which could be self-treated, cost the

NHS an estimated £2 billion every year. Many of these can be treated just as effectively by over-the-counter medications from your local pharmacy, saving you time and money.

However, making the decision to see your GP isn't always clear cut, and you should never put off seeing your doctor if you're concerned about any aspect of your health, no matter how insignificant it might seem. Sometimes minor complaints can turn out to be more serious, so it's important to become aware of your own body, what's normal and be alert to any unusual symptoms.

"Most GPs are wonderful, but we're not experts in every condition," explains Dr Paul Ettlinger, private GP and Founder of the London

General Practice, which is associated with the London Clinic: *www.thelondonclinic.co.uk.* "Don't be frightened to ask for a referral to a specialist. It's important to catch things early on, as treatment is usually more successful. If a problem doesn't go away or you're still worried, go back and ask for a second opinion. Be persistent and mention every new symptom. Think about working 'with' your GP in partnership and be the champion of your own health.

"A trusting relationship with your doctor, where you can be open and honest, is

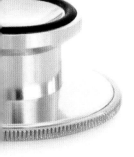

> **You can discuss anything with your GP in complete confidence, so try not to feel embarrassed; your doctor will have seen it all before**

Talk to your GP about what's recommended for you. Some screening tests, such as those for bowel, cervical and breast cancers, and abdominal aortic aneurysms (AAA) are part of a nationwide programme in the UK. If you're offered a screening test, it's important to take it up, as treatment is more likely to be successful if a condition is caught early on.

"Of course, prevention is key," concludes Dr Ettlinger. "I offer a variety of screening tests, and with my patients over 50 years old I undertake a variety of blood tests, cervical smear, mammogram, PSA, chest CT, coronary calcium score, carotid doppler test, a dexa scan and full physical examination. Careful interpretation of these results is, of course, important, but if conditions can be caught early then treatment if far more likely to be successful."

vitally important," continues Dr Ettlinger. "You can discuss anything with your GP in complete confidence, so try not to feel embarrassed; your doctor will have seen it all before."

Prevention

Your GP is also there to offer health checks, and various screening and medical tests, depending on your age, family history, risk factors and gender.

MAKING YOUR APPOINTMENT

1 Is it appropriate to see your GP for your ailment? Should you go to A&E, your local pharmacy, minor injuries unit or just stay at home with self care? Do you have a musculoskeletal problem that a physiotherapist could treat?
If unsure, contact NHS Direct: www.nhsdirect.nhs.uk or dial 111.

2 Make a list of your symptoms and be specific, making a note of when they started and what makes things better or worse.

3 Prepare for your appointment. Take a list of questions and think about what you want to ask your doctor.

4 Take a notepad and write down what your doctor says. Ask them to repeat anything you're not sure about and for an explanation of words that you do not understand or need made clearer.

5 Be clear about what you want your doctor to do, such as refer you to a specialist or change your medication. Be assertive, but polite.

6 Talk to the receptionist about your problem when booking your appointment. You may be able to see the practice nurse instead.

7 You can take a friend or relative to your appointment if you're anxious and to help you remember what the doctor's said during your visit.

8 If you're prescribed any medication or treatment, double check the dose and instructions before you leave.

9 Avoid telling your GP what you think is wrong with you, armed with research from the internet. Let them reach their own diagnosis.

10 Mention all medication and supplements, herbal or homeopathic remedies that you take.

Health round-up

Getting a good night's sleep is one of the best things you can do for your health and is a basic human need. Yet, 47% of us claim we're too stressed to sleep, and a worrying number of people survive on only five or six hours per night.

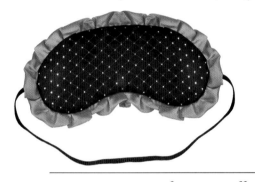

42% of women suffer in silence because pelvic floor health is a hugely overlooked subject. It's estimated that it can take women up to ten years to seek help for problems such as urine incontinence and prolapse. Help is available and you shouldn't suffer in silence. Don't be embarrassed to talk to your doctor.

Constipation affects one in five people over the age of 65 and can seriously affect health and quality of life. Don't be embarrassed to talk about your bowel health, especially if you notice unusual bleeding. See your GP for help.

Diabetes is the UK's biggest health concern, accounting for 10% of the entire NHS budget, and is a time bomb with serious consequences. Reduce your chances of developing it by being as active as you can, eating a healthy diet and losing weight.

BE AWARE OF HOW YOUR BODY WORKS and, if things change or you notice unusual symptoms, make an appointment to see your GP. Don't bury your head in the sand or ignore problems. Many diseases can be treated more successfully if found early.

Cigarette smoking is the single cause of preventable death in the UK. Give up, and within ten years your risk of lung cancer has fallen to around half that of a smoker. www. quit.org.uk

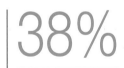

38% of all cancers are preventable with healthy lifestyle choices, better diet and weight management. Find out more at *www.wcrf.org.uk.*

80% of us have gum disease. If you have gum disease, you're three times more likely to have a heart attack. Cleaning between your teeth every day is almost more important than brushing. See your dentist if you notice bleeding gums.

Final word
Not all health conditions are totally preventable, but there's a lot we can all do to reduce our risk of developing various diseases and cancer. Take control, be proactive and responsible for your own health. Your future health is in your hands.

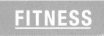

'Fit is not a destination, it's a way of life'

Anon

Embrace
fitness

You might still feel 21 at heart, but your body might not agree. Like it or not, our bodies change as we get older. From around the age of 40, we begin to lose muscle, our cardiovascular fitness declines, and we can become less flexible and lose mobility. But while we can't totally prevent these inevitable physiological changes, there's a huge amount we can do to slow them down and stay as fit, healthy and strong as possible.
- Be inspired!

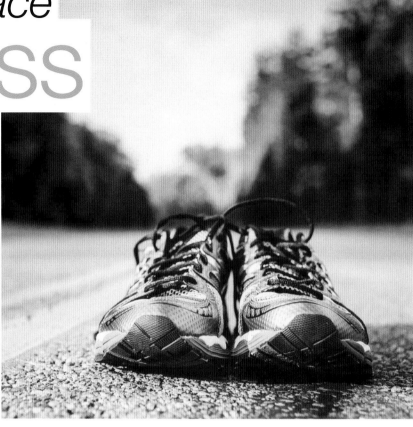

CASE STUDY IMAGE: 'CASTLE TRIATHLON SERIES'

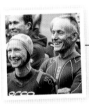

Jo & Paul's Story

Jo Clift, 51, and husband Paul, 61, compete in long-distance triathlon, running and swimming events. Their story shows that anything's possible

"Having been fairly active, but a long way from athletic, we took up running two weeks before Paul's 56th birthday. Our challenge was whether we could run to the end of the road and back. Within six months, we were running half marathons, and in 18 months we completed the Swiss Alpine 50-mile ultra marathon. Jo then decided she wanted to learn to swim properly, and we found ourselves in the novice lane of a local triathlon club. With some experience of social cycling, we completed a sprint distance triathlon four months later.

"Within three years, we completed Iron Distance triathlons (which involve a 2.4-mile swim, 112-mile bike and full marathon) and long-distance open-water swim events up to 10K, becoming (age category) National Champions at both distances and representing Great Britain in the World Olympic distance triathlon championships along the way. We've loved every minute of our 'journey'!"

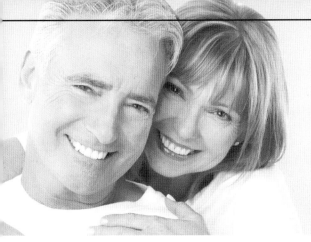

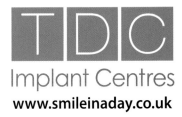

Implant Centres

www.smileinaday.co.uk

The ultimate alternative to dentures

"**Everybody is saying how beautiful my new teeth look!**"

Sally Ann - Smile In A Day patient

"Such a professional team. I felt in very good hands."

Gerard - Smile In A Day patient

Award Winning* Dental Implant Treatment. No more loose, missing or false teeth

Before

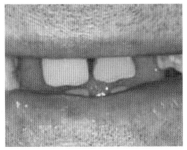

After

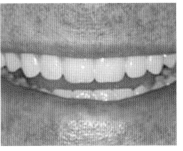

Call today to arrange your **free, no obligation** consultation.

0800 041 3028**

Visit our website for more info:
www.smileinaday.co.uk

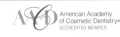

Effects
of ageing

Maintaining muscle mass and bone density through exercise can offset some of the effects of ageing, such as sarcopenia, osteoporosis and weight gain

Muscle loss

The medical term sarcopenia refers to the loss of muscle mass and strength that occurs with ageing. It's a complex process and is usually seen in inactive people, worsening over the age of 70 years. Dietary and hormonal factors also play a part in the development of the disease.

Research conducted on astronauts – who also suffer muscle mass loss due to low gravity and inactivity – found that resistance training and increased dietary protein were key in preventing and, in some cases, reversing sarcopenia.

Did you know?

A recent report in the BMJ analysed hundreds of trials involving 340,000 patients, and found that physical activity was as effective as medication in managing conditions such as heart disease, stroke and pre-diabetes.

In a study in the USA, elderly people who did 45 minutes of resistance training three times a week for 12 weeks saw a 30% increase in muscle strength.

In another study in 2011, athletes aged 40-81 years, who exercised four to five times a week, showed results indicating that both muscle mass and strength were maintained across the ages. (see the cross-section image of the thigh on the opposite page).

Cardiovascular changes

Your heart rate slows by around one beat per year from birth, and maximum aerobic capacity starts to decline from the age of 40. If the heart muscle also gets weaker due to a lack of exercise or

METABOLIC DECREASE

According to the National Obesity Forum, having a waist measurement of more than 35" for women and 40" for men represents a "substantially increased risk" of developing heart disease, stroke, some cancers and Type-2 diabetes.

Your basal metabolic rate is thought to decrease by around 1-2% per decade. If, for example, your energy requirements were 2200kcal per day in your 30s, by the time you're over 50 you could need 200kcal per day less. It might not seem a lot, but over time – and without enough physical activity – it will lead to an inevitable fat gain and change in body composition. If, however, you lead an active lifestyle and do resistance training to maintain muscle mass, you can offset the majority of this metabolic decrease.

is less efficient due to blood vessels being blocked by fatty deposits, it doesn't pump blood and oxygen around the body as well. Like muscle loss, however, a decline in aerobic capacity isn't inevitable and there's a lot you can do to keep your heart healthy.

Bone density

Loss of bone density, known as osteoporosis, can develop as we get older, leading to weak bones and fractures. From the age of 35, we're all prone to losing bone mass, but the losses differ from individual to individual, depending on age,

activity levels, diet and family history. Weight-bearing activity such as running, walking, dancing and weight training can help to maintain bone density and slow down the rate of loss as we age (see p28 for more on osteoporosis).

Weight gain

Losing muscle mass has the effect of reducing metabolism. Eat the same amount of food as you did in your 30s, in conjunction with being less active, and you have a recipe for weight gain, in particular an increase in abdominal fat around the waistline.

AGEING MUSCLES

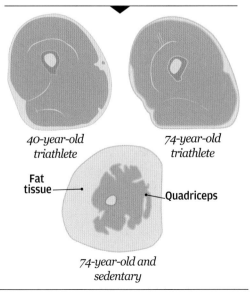

40-year-old triathlete

74-year-old triathlete

Fat tissue

Quadriceps

74-year-old and sedentary

Exercise
priorities

Physical activity is, without doubt, the most important thing you can do as you get older. Keeping your body strong, fit and healthy will give you a fighting chance of not just living longer, but avoiding many preventable illnesses and conditions

But what do we mean by "physical activity"? While a stroll to the shops is a great way to stay active, it's probably not enough to offset the effects of ageing or make much difference to your cardiovascular function or muscle mass.

We're talking about exercise. The sort of exercise that raises your heart rate and gets you breathless. The sort that keeps your muscles strong and flexible, and your body toned. And the sort that will help you to stay active, mobile and healthy well into your 70s, 80s and beyond.

> *Fitness needs to become a lifestyle, not a chore. It can be hard to get started or back into if you haven't been active for a while*

Muscle loss

Preventing muscle loss and strength is the main priority for anyone over 50. Do it with some kind of resistance training – using weights in the gym, or a circuit class or some sort of home workout using weights, bands or body weight exercises – or a class such as bodypump or TRX. Sports such as swimming and rowing, which incorporate some sort of resistance can be good, too. Running and walking are great for all-round fitness, but won't build specific strength.

ACSM Guidelines (2009) recommend "older athletes" do two to three "resistance training" sessions per week, incorporating two to three sets of 8-12 repetitions of each exercise. This could be

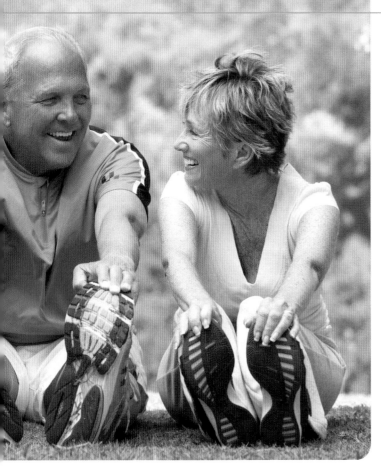

Think of your fitness programme as a jigsaw puzzle made up of four main pieces:

❶ LIFESTYLE ACTIVITY
Just move more. Walk as much as you can for transport and avoid taking the car. Activities such as gardening and housework all count as lifestyle activity, too.

❷ RESISTANCE TRAINING
Building and maintaining muscle and strength is a priority. Circuit or weight training – 20 minutes of exercises two to three times a week – is easily done at home.

❸ AGILITY, BALANCE AND CO-ORDINATION
Maintain these important aspects of fitness to prevent falls and stay agile with a mixture of activities such as dancing, fitness classes, running and games like badminton.

❹ CARDIOVASCULAR FITNESS
Do specific aerobic exercise where you get your heart rate up for a consistent time. Jogging, cycling, dancing, football… anything that gets you out of breath.

◀ IN A NUTSHELL, IT'S SIMPLE
Aim to move more. Avoid sitting in front of the TV or computer for long periods of time. Think about your lifestyle and how you could incorporate activity in other, more innovative ways. If you enjoy listening to music, could you do it while walking instead of sitting at home? Could you ride your bike to work or the shops instead of taking the car? Waiting for the kettle to boil? Then you have time to do a couple of sets of squats.

done at home with a range of equipment, taking only 20-30 minutes (see p82 on getting the best from a home gym).

Aerobic capacity

Cardiovascular exercise keeps your heart and lungs healthy, and helps to maintain aerobic capacity. But it needs to get your heart rate up, and for you to feel breathless and sweaty.

NHS guidelines suggest that "older adults aged 65 or older, who are generally fit and have no health conditions, should try to be active daily and should do at least 150 minutes (two hours and 30 minutes) of moderate-intensity aerobic activity such as cycling or fast walking every week". Although that sound a lot, when broken down it's around 20 minutes a day, and even more achievable if you break it up into 10-minute chunks.

Fitness needs to become a lifestyle, not a chore. But it can be hard to get started or back into it if you haven't been active for a while. Our modern-day energy-saving environment doesn't make it easy for us to be active, so it needs to be a conscious decision.

Are you active enough?

70% *of us say we want to be more physically active, but we claim to have too many work commitments and a lack of leisure time, according to a report published by the British Heart Foundation*

But are we being honest with ourselves?

With the average Brit reported to spend 20 hours a day sleeping, lying down or sitting, we're risking our health by being inactive. We can't continue to make excuses, says the World Heart Foundation (WHF), which is urging people to be more self-aware and start moving.

Become more aware

One in three people questioned by the WHF had no idea how active they are. Awareness is the first step in making a change. Find out exactly how active you are (or not) by wearing a pedometer, such as a Fitbug. It can be a big wake-up call, as most people significantly overestimate their activity level. Simply wearing a pedometer can encourage you to be more active, too. A recent study showed an increase in physical activity of 26.9% by using a pedometer.

There's strong evidence that exercising reduces your risk of chronic diseases and improves your quality of life. New research involving over 55s confirms exercising and losing weight as the most effective treatments for osteoarthritis.

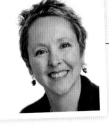

Alisa's Story

Alisa was diagnosed with breast cancer at the age of 42

"Becoming healthier is about the little choices I can make in the present moment. It's the decision right in front of me about what I'll eat today; whether I'll walk, ride my bike, or get some other exercise; what time I go to bed; and every other choice that makes a difference to my health."

Getting started

Making a conscious choice to improve your quality of life through health and fitness is the first step. But don't rely on willpower or just hoping it will happen. You have to take control and make it work for you.

The next step is to get organised. Plan and structure your fitness schedule and activities to suit your lifestyle. There are endless ways to exercise. Be realistic and think about your personality; your likes and dislikes; whether you are a team player or prefer exercising alone (complete the quiz on p66). And stick with it, says Prof Steve Peters, consultant psychiatrist working in sport and author of *The Chimp Paradox*: "When planning, take into account the ways in which you're likely to sabotage your own progress or commitment (look back to past experience for evidence). Work out what encourages you to keep going and monitor that."

TOP TIPS

Starting out and staying on track

1 Map out your fitness schedule and keep it visible.

2 Make exercise a priority. Don't just wait until you have time.

3 Be organised: book activities and classes into your schedule.

4 Consider home workouts such as yoga, weights, toning stretching and dancing. Mowing the lawn counts.

5 Join a group to help you persevere when it gets tough.

Kim's Story

Kim, 54 mum of 4, from London

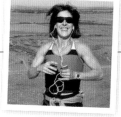

"I used what I called the 'mini portion approach', first developed when I had lots of young children! No amount of time was too small to squeeze in something. Sometimes, I just had three minutes to pull six dandelions out of the garden, or grab a skipping rope and do five minutes before my screaming child needed me. But in this way, the garden bloomed and I got fitter.

"It's about baby steps. Get into your fitness kit first thing in the morning; it signifies intent and commitment. Never make up or wash before exercise, as there's something inhibiting about having to redo it! "

Small strides towards fitness

The Fitbug is a wearable fitness tracker complete with a coaching plan that provides progress reports and sets regular goals to keep you on track: *www.fitbug.com*

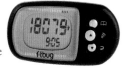

Setting
goals

Find your mojo

What is it you really want? This key question is your starting point. "To make positive and long-term change that resonates, you need to be committed to, not just interested in, achieving goals," says Alison Forge, mentor and author of *Pocket Positivity*, who helps people through the process of making life changes.

Write a list of things that you'd like to achieve and be realistic. Start by making a few small changes, and you'll soon feel your confidence grow and your purpose become stronger as you tick off each goal. Focus on "today" rather than the outcome of "running a 45-minute 10km within two months". Goals include signing up to a cycling group or yoga class; meeting a friend for a walk; even waking up in a positive mood and doing 10 minutes of stretching before you start your day.

Results *are* rewards

A recent study found that 25% of people gained weight once they joined the gym, as they give themselves treats after a workout. See the reward in the healthy lifestyle changes you've made instead of "a gift" for yourself after exercising. Feeling fitter, sleeping better, laughing more – these are rewards. Enjoying a spin class, or feeling a buzz all day after an early morning run are your rewards.

What the experts say

"Having goals that are clear, realistic and measurable is crucial. The core factor is that goals must be meaningful and consistent, with self-endorsed values rather than being made on a whim or as a result of New Year resolutions, for example, where you say to yourself, 'I should exercise more'.

"You have to believe in yourself and really know how you're going to achieve your

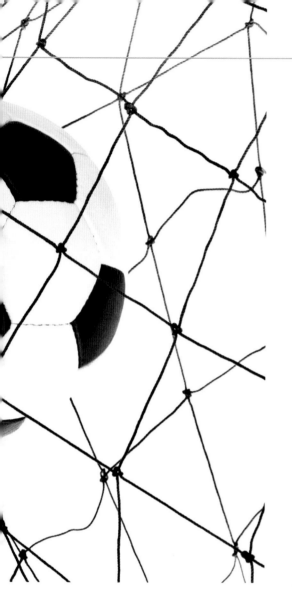

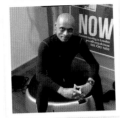

Morris's Story

Morris Tolaram, 55, weight trains and runs regularly

"While age can impact all fitness components, we can still improve fitness levels by taking advantage of our experience, patience and smarter training regimes. As I get older, to stay injury free I extend my warm-ups, warm-downs and flexibility component. I've learned from previous injuries, and alter my programme or rest if I have a niggle."

TOP TIPS

❶ You may find it motivating to work towards a goal - your local charity walk or 5km run can be a great target.

❷ Make the most of your gym membership with classes and sessions, and attend one or two each week to build up consistency.

❸ Commit to meeting a friend for a game of squash or tennis, and be sure to turn up!

❹ If you love the outdoors, buy some OS maps and plan solo/group walks, or go trail running.

❺ Allow yourself rest days to stay injury free.

❻ Blend your new fitness regime into your lifestyle, and make it fun and social.

❼ Get your family and friends on board – support speaks in volumes.

---

goals. You have to believe you can do it. You must explore you own reasons for changing in order to be fully committed to making a change. These key questions are based on outcome expectancies and self-efficacy, such as 'how confident am I?'. Ask yourself, 'what is it I really want?'"
Martin S Hagger, PhD, Professor of Psychology, Curtin University, Perth, Australia

Pull it all together

❯ Step 1 Awareness. How active are you? Be honest about your likes and dislikes, too.

❯ Step 2 Get organised and plan what you're going to do.

❯ Step 3 Put it into practice and focus on the rewards of a healthy lifestyle.

❯ Step 4 Sustain your positive and new lifestyle changes.

Make it work for you

"Get the right team around you. Fill your life with energy givers; the ones who always enthuse and encourage you. Consider not just the physical or practical aspects of what you want to achieve, but also the emotional aspects and what is reasonable for you." *Professor Steve Peters, who supported the British cycling team at London 2012 Olympics*

What's right for you?

Finding an activity you enjoy is the key to lifelong exercise.
It doesn't matter whether it's dancing, cycling or pilates
– if it works for you then that's all that matters

How would your friends describe you?

A Focused and determined. When you set a goal, there's no stopping you.

B Giving and caring, but you can lack confidence.

C Spontaneous and a free spirit.

D Life and soul of the party!

How do you cope with a stressful day?

A Go out for a brisk jog.

B Settle down on the sofa with a cup of tea.

C Clear your head with an evening stroll.

D Head to the pub to meet friends.

Do you set New Year resolutions?

A Yes, but I'm constantly setting goals all year round.

B Every year, then feel despondent by February when I've given up,

C No. I'm happy with my life and have no need to change it.

D I prefer to make a list of goals and plans.

Did you enjoy sport at school?

A Yes, I was competitive and quite good.

B No, I was always picked last for teams.

C Preferred doing activities with my family.

D I liked team games such as hockey or netball.

What's your ideal holiday?

A Pack in as much as possible. Sightseeing, sunbathing, hiking and squeeze in a few work emails, too.

B Relaxing at a villa with a pool, a quiet beach and a good book.

C A walking holiday in the mountains or coastal paths.

D With friends. Maybe a cruise with nice restaurants and good nightlife.

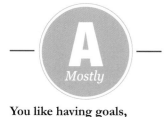

A — Mostly

You like having goals, getting results, and need routine and rules to function at your best. You're committed and disciplined.

You need activity with a purpose, so try cycling, running, swimming lengths or hiking, and work on setting achieveable goals, such as a local 10km. Pilates or yoga, which require focus and self-control, will provide some balance.

Avoid sticking with the plan at all costs. Maintain perspective and allow yourself rest days when you're tired or ill.

B — Mostly

You have good intentions, but struggle to get started. Finding the time to exercise is hard, as there's always something better to do. A previous experience may have put you off and you can feel self-conscious. You feel uncomfortable getting out of breath, hot and sweaty.

You need classes and sessions fixed in your diary. Don't set your goals too high or try anything too tough – keep it easy and fun. Aerobics, Zumba, Nordic walking, jogging or cycling groups would all be great choices. Arrange to meet a friend for a walk or game of tennis, and don't back out!

Avoid home exercise DVDs or solo exercise, which just sets you up for failure. You need social interaction, structure and pre-booked commitments.

C — Mostly

You love nature, spontaneity, feeling free and fresh air. You don't like gyms, exercise to music classes or bootcamps. You like to exercise when you feel like it and you use exercise to relieve stress.

You need to focus on enjoyment and being at one with nature. You may enjoy the mind-body interaction of pilates and yoga. Natural activities such as hiking, trail running, cycling, horse riding or wild swimming will appeal to you.

Avoid being alone, too, all the time. Social interaction is important. Once in a while, meet up with a friend for a bike ride, or try joining a friendly jogging group, horse riding with a friend or walking club.

D — Mostly

You enjoy the company of others and love a good gossip. You're sociable, full of life and fun to be with. You get bored exercising on your own and rely on the support of others to keep you motivated.

You need social interaction. Choose exercise groups with other people, where you can make friends and catch up for a chat. You'll probably enjoy most types of exercise so long as you're with friends, so try cycling groups, rambling, dancing and racquet games. Keep things fun and you'll reap the rewards.

Avoid putting pressure on yourself to achieve goals or targets, and try not to get too competitive with your friends. Just have fun. Avoid home exercise or going it alone, too.

Get into...
walking

Walking can easily be integrated into your daily routine, either as a simple mode of transport or a brisk walk with the dog. Or how about joining a local rambling group?

Walking is one of the most simple, yet effective forms of exercise. You can do it with friends, alone or with your dog. It can be long and leisurely or brisk and short. It can be something you do for fitness, or just as a way of getting to work or the shops.

Our expert says

"Walking is something you can do at any age and is easily integrated into your daily routine, so you're much more likely to enjoy it and do it regularly. It can work for anyone, whether you're looking for vigorous exercise or a more gentle pace."
Joanna Hall MSc, Diet and Movement Expert

Consistent walking can be a really powerful form of exercise for lifelong health, and can be more effective than

Find out more about the Walkactive technique by Joanna Hall at *www. joannahall.com*. Try the Walkactive Starter Pack, which includes an instructional DVD, book and pedometer.

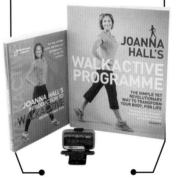

short-term intense bursts of exercise or short-lived gym membership. Think of it as a lifestyle.

In a study of 70,000 female nurses, it was found that those who walked at a brisk pace on most days of the week for at least 30 minutes reduced their risk of stroke by 40%.

Benefits of walking

The benefits of walking are endless. Improved posture, reduced back pain, weight loss, reduced blood pressure and cholesterol, stress relief and better cardiovascular fitness, to mention just a few. And as a weight-bearing exercise, walking is one of the best forms of exercise to help maintain bone density, so ideal if you're concerned about or suffer from osteoporosis.

How to do it?

▸ Specific fitness walking: start gradually with 10-minute walks and build from there. It's better to do a short, brisk walk every day. Aim for consistency and regularity.

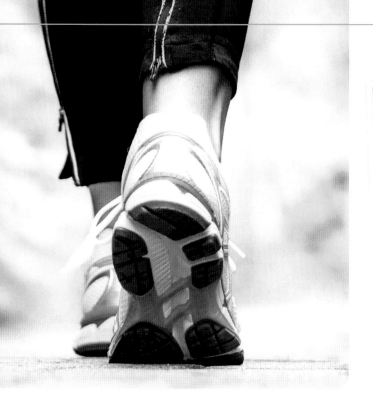

Liz's Story

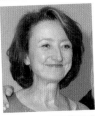

Liz from London walks every day for fitness

"I hate any form of exercise, but walking I do on my own. I try to do a walk every day and use the Joanna Hall Walkactive method. I feel empowered. It's made me feel better, friends say I look fantastic and my stress has gone. If I wake up feeling lousy, I know after a walk I'll feel much better. I'm very pleased with myself and can't recommend Walkactive highly enough for ladies of a certain age."

▶ As a simple mode of transport: walk to work, or part of the way by getting off the bus earlier or parking the car further away. Leave the car at home and walk to the shops for your daily paper.

▶ Try a rambling group for a long, leisurely stroll: *www.ramblers.org.uk*

▶ Nordic walking provides an all-over body workout. By incorporating walking poles, you use your upper body. Find your local class: *www.nordicwalking.co.uk*

▶ Try the free Health Walk Scheme: *www.walkingforhealth. org.uk*

▶ Get an active dog! They need walking every day and can't be ignored.

SIGN UP FOR A WALKING CHALLENGE

MOONWALK
Walk a half, full or ultra marathon through the streets of London or in Scotland at night to raise money for and awareness of breast cancer. For more information, go to *www.walkthewalk.org*
Or, to experience a once-in-a-lifetime trip to stunning locations such as Machu Picchu or Everest Base Camp, try a sponsored trek with *www.action.org.uk*

MERRELL ACCESS ARC
GREAT FOR POWER WALKING WITH ITS LOW PROFILE AND WIDE TOE BOX

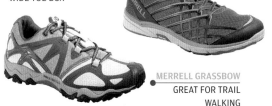

MERRELL GRASSBOW
GREAT FOR TRAIL WALKING

WHAT TYPE OF FOOTWEAR?

Invest in the right footwear for the terrain you'll be walking on and the type of walking you'll be doing. Trainers or lightweight trekking shoes are best for brisk power walking; traditional boots are better for rambling and hill walking. Choose a shoe with a wide toebox, which allows the toes and foot to spread and move freely. Try a specific walking shoe such as the Merrell: *www.merrell.co.uk*

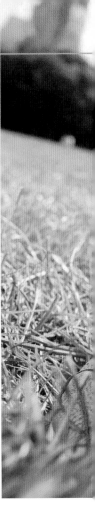

Get into...
running

Running is one of the best forms of cardiovascular exercise, reducing your risk of heart disease, diabetes, hypertension, cancer and much, much more

Running also helps with depression, weight control, muscle strength, mobility and balance, and is also a great way to keep your bones strong. As we get older, these benefits are increased, so there are even more reasons to keep running as long as you can.

Age is no barrier

In the 2013 Virgin London Marathon, almost 15% of the participants were over the age of 50. And performance doesn't have to suffer, either. In 2012, British marathon runner Dave Cartwright ran two hours, 54 minutes to win the over-60 age category – a time most runners half his age can only dream of.

Concerns for older people

Physiological changes mean that older runners do need more rest and recovery time, especially after races or hard runs. Pay more attention to your diet, eating more protein, and focus on recovery nutrition with a post-run recovery shake.

Staying on track

It's thought that 82% of runners get injured every year and the risk is higher for older runners. Incorporate regular strength and conditioning sessions at least twice a week, and get a regular sports massage. New research also suggests older runners should only run three times a week, and spend more time cross training to avoid injury.

Adapt your running to suit your time of life. If you've been competitive in the past, it might be time to focus on a different distance or switch to trail running or relay events. And rather than compare yourself against old times, focus on your position within your age group or your age-graded percentage.

What about arthritis?

Contrary to popular belief, running doesn't cause arthritis. The National Runners' Health Study in the US recently (2013) published data that showed runners are actually half as likely to develop osteoarthritis or to need a hip or knee replacement

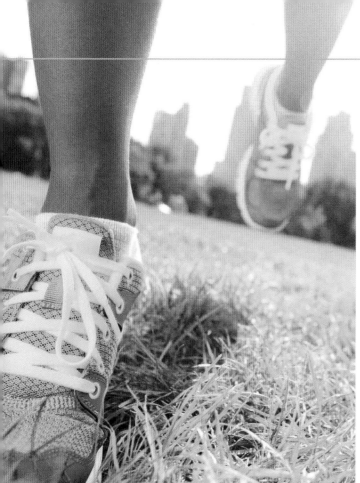

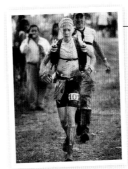

Mimi's Story

Mimi Anderson, 51, is the UK's most decorated female ultra runner and holder of multiple Guinness World Records

"I'd never been very sporty and only started running in my late 30s. I did a 5km and was hooked! I realised that although I wasn't very fast, I could keep going for long distances. In 2001, I entered the Marathon des Sables (156 miles across the Sahara) and I fell in love with crazy, long distances, setting records and attempting things other people didn't think were possible. I've set three World Records including running 345 miles from North to South Ireland and John O'Groats to Lands End.

"I love the freedom running gives me, the space to be by myself and to experience stunning places I'd never otherwise see. For years, I suffered with anorexia and running has helped me overcome it, get back my confidence and be stronger.

"As well as running, I do a lot of strength work in the gym. As I get older, I need to do more of it to stay strong and injury free. Just running isn't enough. I worry about osteoporosis, but running helps keeps my bones strong, too.

"I know what I do is fairly extreme, but I believe you can do anything you set your mind to and age isn't a barrier. I hope to be running and setting records into my 70s and beyond."
www.marvellousmimi.com

compared to walkers. Instead of wearing joints down, in healthy and previously uninjured runners it appears that running can actually strengthen them.

Our expert says

"I think that once you get past the age of 65, your main thought should be on staying fit and healthy, and living a long and healthy life. You do have to spend more time on warming up and cooling down, and look after yourself between runs. Keep running as long as you can."

Bruce Tulloh, former International runner and author of Running Over Forty.

How to get started

If you're brand new to running, try a complete beginner jog/walk plan such as the NHS Couch to 5km plan. Check out your local Run England beginner group for supervision and support: *www.runengland.org*

You're never too old to take up running, but make sure you get a check-up from your doctor before you start.

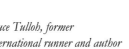

Get into...
cycling

It can be hard to get started if you've never ridden a bike before or if the last time was 30 years ago. But it's worth persevering, as cycling is a fantastic sport for people of all ages

Cycling is excellent for your health. It gets you outdoors, and it's great for your cardiovascular fitness and leg strength, not to mention your mental health, wellbeing and sense of freedom.

Using your bike as a mode of transport to visit friends, pop to the shops or to and from work is also a clever way to fit exercise into your busy lifestyle. It's also a great alternative to running and can result in less injury risk.

Research says
A study by the University of Sydney in 2013 found that people aged 49-79, who had cycled in the preceding month, performed significantly better on decision time and response time tests, and those who cycled at least an hour a week showed significant improvements in balance.

Build it up
Start slowly and build up the length of time you ride for. Try including some additional leg strength training (squats and lunges), which will benefit your cycling, too. Make sure you're comfortable on the bike (consider a professional bike fit), and you can then build up your distances quite quickly, working up to an hour or two at a steady pace.

Breeze rides
British Cycling has come up with a great solution for women with its newly launched women-only Breeze Cycling Groups (*www. goskyride.com/breeze*), which are available nationwide. Rides are led by trained female ride leaders, are aimed at complete novice women riders, and held on mostly traffic-free, quiet roads.

Where to ride?
There are lots of traffic-free cycle routes, such as old railway lines, canal paths and forest trails, all over the UK, which are ideal if you're

TOP TIP

Keep your bike well serviced so it's ready to go at all times, and consider attending a cycle maintenance course so you know how to change a tyre or fix a dropped chain

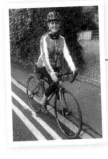

Janice's Story

Janice Bailey, 71, **is a competitive cyclist and rides with a club**

"I bought my first road bike in 2004 aged 63 and started competing in sprint distance triathlons. I graduated to Olympic distance by 2009, but I was advised to give running a miss after some knee trouble. I've gradually stepped up the pace and become more competitive, last year winning our interclub time trial handicap. I get a buzz from hard riding, whether it's racing or hill climbing. It's very satisfying to feel comfortable riding with younger people. My health is excellent with none of the heart and blood pressure problems most of my peer group seems to suffer from. Thank goodness for my bike!" *With thanks to www. kentvelogirls.co.uk*

new to cycling. Have a look at *www.sustrans.org.uk*, the charity behind 12,000 miles of National Cycle Network.

Equipment essentials

Although not compulsory in the UK, a helmet is highly recommended. Make sure it fits well. You'll also need high-visibility or bright clothing, a bell, lock, tool and puncture kit, and lights if riding at night, as well as padded shorts.

Take it more seriously

Joining a club is a great way to get more out of you cycling, and there are over 1500 clubs all over the UK: *www.britishcycling.org.uk*

Try a cyclosportive event, which is an organised and timed ride, but not a race. They are usually low key, relaxed and great fun, and offer a variety of distances and terrains: *www.cyclosport.org*

Our expert says

"When riding on the road, think about using your ears as much as your eyes, and remain vigilant and aware, yet relaxed and confident. It goes without saying that listening to music or wearing headphones isn't advisable." *Kirsti Grayson, British Cycling tutor and Director of cycle training company Go Velo: www.govelo.co.uk*

Road safety

If you're unsure about riding on the road, try attending an adult cycling training course. Courses are available at *www.bikeability.org.uk* and teach a wide range of skills, including basic bike handling and riding in traffic.

Get into...
swimming

Swimming is the perfect cardiovascular and low-impact exercise – a great way to keep active

Swimming can reduce the risk of heart disease, type-2 diabetes and stroke. It's readily accessible, sociable and can be practised all year. It's also a good way to keep active if you have joint mobility problems.

Rejuvenating effects
Research shows swimming boosts your mood and stimulates pulmonary systems. Swimmers typically have stronger muscles with greater endurance and demonstrate better coordination, reducing the risk of injury, improving posture and increasing the ability to perform daily tasks.

Getting started
If you have existing health concerns, see your GP before you start. Visit your local pool for information on classes for your age group and level, and one-to-one lessons; both can help improve your confidence and technique. Go Swimming is a good resource for expert advice and information: *www.swimming.org/go*

Go to the next level
To improve your performance, add some interval sessions to your schedule or join a masters club. Masters offer age group competition, and men and women race separately. Visit British Swimming: *www.swimming.org*

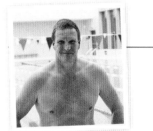

Peter's Story
Peter Morris, 51, **came 4th in the 200m butterfly final at the 1980 Olympic Games**

"I started swimming again about three years ago, and now swim three to four times a week. After quite a few years away from the pool, my motivation in starting again was to get fitter and keep the weight off. It's also social, and gives me the chance to chat with regulars and have a laugh. Swimming is an excellent way of maintaining a good level of fitness and protecting your joints, and helping you sleep and eat well. I feel a real buzz after a session!"

Spice it up
Read up and incorporate strength and mobilising exercises, static stretches and developmental stretches to complement your swimming.

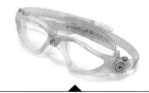

TRY THESE:
AQUA SPHERE KAYENNE GOGGLES
WWW.AQUASPHERESWIM.COM/UK

Get into...
triathlon

Triathlon is the fastest growing sport in the UK, and a fantastic choice for older people

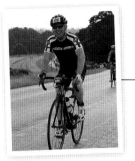

Triathlon is accessible to everyone, regardless of age or ability, and is a great choice for older competitors due to the balance of training for three different sports. The combination of swimming, running and cycling develops both upper and lower body strength and good cardiovascular endurance. It also reduces risk of injury when compared to a single sport such as running.

Getting started

A typical sprint triathlon is usually 400m swim, 20km bike ride and 5km run, although shorter novice distances are popular, too. You don't need to be super fit or have expensive equipment. You can take part with an old mountain bike and get by with any swimming stroke that works for you. You can train for a triathlon with one session per sport each week – start gradually and build up each discipline.

Events are open to beginners, women and people of all ages, and can be in a swimming pool, lake or river or through woods or on a trail. Find out more at *www.britishtriathlon.org*

The next level

The beauty of triathlon is the focus on competition within your age group rather than overall position or time. Age groups are five years apart, so there's a great opportunity to do well at local events. It's even possible to qualify for Team GB at 'Age Group' World or European Championships for age groups right up to 80 years old. Ironman and long-distance triathlons are also becoming more popular and appeal to older athletes who generally have better endurance.

Our expert says

"Over the last 12 months, we've seen a 25% growth in people over 50 taking part in

Steve's Story

Steve Archbold, 56 from Kent, is a police officer and competes in triathlons

"I've always had to maintain a level of fitness for my job, but as I got older I found that I was picking up injuries from running. I thought triathlon would provide an all-round fitness and might be fun.

"I bought my first road bike at 53. I'm not a great swimmer, but it doesn't matter as I can make it up on the bike and run. I enjoy the variety of training, and find that mixing up running, cycling and swimming keeps me motivated and provides a well-rounded training regime."

our triathlons. In fact, the over 50s is the biggest growing age group, which shows that triathlon is a fantastic sport for older people."
Brian Adcock, organiser of the Castle Triathlon Series, www.castletriathlonseries.co.uk

Get into...
racquet sports

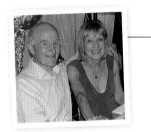

A regular game of squash, tennis or badminton can help keep your muscles strong and flexible

Badminton

Badminton is a great way to keep your entire body strong and supple. Include stretching and conditioning exercises to avoid injury and allow your body to adjust to the increase in range of movement: *www.badmintonengland.co.uk*

▶ Our expert says

"Badminton is a fantastic sport for the over 50s because it offers everything from social participation with friends to world-level competitive events for veterans players." *George Wood, Director of Development, Badminton England*

Squash

Squash is great for your fitness and strength, but it can be intense and is fast moving, so build up slowly if you haven't played for a while. Play with a partner of a similar fitness level *www. englandsquashandracketball.com*

▶ Our expert says

"Squash develops strength and flexibility, as it forces you to increase your range of movement." *Rory Pennell, squash coach, Virgin Active*

Tennis

Tennis improves your anaerobic and aerobic fitness, tones your muscles and works on your balance.

▶ Our expert says

"Tennis helps with flexibility and agility – important for those over 50. It's low impact and brilliant for leg strength, being quick on your feet and fast bursts of energy." *Steve*

Bill's Story

Bill Boylett, 74, **played for England in the World Senior Badminton Championships in 2013**

"Playing badminton has had a huge effect on my life. My father was a smoker and died at 55, so I've never smoked and always been active and maintained a healthy diet. I've also recently started using beetroot juice, which has made me feel fantastic.

"After being made redundant, I started playing badminton to help relieve stress, and I got better and joined a club. It was a turning point in my life. I couldn't wait for the next match. My wife and I have met over a thousand people through badminton." *With thanks to www.beet-it.com*

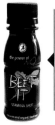

BILL USES BEET IT TO HELP WITH HIS PERFORMANCE. BEET IT IS SHOWN TO IMPROVE ENDURANCE PERFORMANCE BY 15% AND REDUCE BLOOD PRESSURE.

Get into...
golfing

Golf is a fantastic social sport that's good for your health and your heart. An 18-hole course provides about four miles of rigorous walking in the great outdoors, giving you plenty of fresh air and access to Vitamin D

Better with age

The number of people over 65 playing golf is increasing dramatically, according to surveys by Sport England, with more women taking it up for the first time, too. Regular golfers happily spend five hours at a weekend enjoying a leisurely game. Playing regularly helps you stay mobile, and improve your muscle tone and endurance.

Our expert says

"People often question the fitness and health benefits of golf. However, research has demonstrated that playing 18 holes of golf three times per week improves cardiovascular fitness and decreases heart disease (if you walk). Golf gets the body moving by taking the joints and muscles through range of motion, improving flexibility while keeping the bones and muscles strong. The best thing about golf is the ability to play and enjoy the game at all ages, from nine to 90 years. You can play with, and compete with, your parent or even your grandparent!"
Rod Hidlebaugh, Physiotherapist and Director, Townsville Clinic, Australia

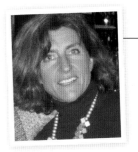

Antonia's Story
Antonia Edgerton, 52, took up golf in 2011

"I first played golf over 20 years ago, but as I didn't take lessons I just hacked around. A couple of years ago, I gave it another shot and really started enjoying it, and I'm constantly improving.

"Golf is something I can do with my husband, either at home or on weekends away. It's great because it's something we do together, sometimes with another couple or in a group. There's also a huge social aspect to playing, with drinks and regular events outside the club to attend. I've seen some beautiful countryside and different terrain."

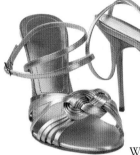

Get into...
dancing

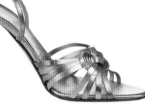

We all love to dance, and the wide variety of options and styles available make it a great activity for everyone, young and old. It can be as

do it, it can be an excellent cardiovascular workout, too. Most importantly, dancing is one of the most fun and sociable ways to stay active.

classes nationwide. Or look in your local paper or community magazine.

Fitness classes

Dance-fused fitness classes such as Zumba are becoming very popular and offer a great blend of aerobic exercise and dance moves. Check out your local leisure centre or gym for classes.

> " *Dance is a great weight-bearing exercise - it's invigorating, engaging and exciting and, most importantly, it appeals to everyone* "

Craig Revel Horwood, TV Dance Judge

vigorous or gentle as you wish. And thanks to popular TV shows, dancing has become one of the fastest growing art forms in the UK. More than 4.8 million people attend community-based dance groups in England each year.

Benefits

From a fitness perspective, dancing keeps you active, improves balance, posture and co-ordination, and as a weight-bearing activity it's great for bone health. Depending on the style and how vigorously you

Getting started

Ballroom dancing has made a comeback in recent years and it can be a great way to meet people or try out a new activity with your partner. Styles such as salsa, tango and ceroc are vibrant, fun and sociable. You could even try more exotic styles such as flamenco, pole dancing or belly dancing. The choice is endless. Try a few different styles and classes to see what you enjoy.

Find a class or instructor at *www.dancenearyou.co.uk*, which has a database of over 1000

"Dancing is a great way of exercising: it's fun, it keeps you fit, improves your balance and really does help to keep your bones healthy."
Moira Holmes, Tea Dance Organiser, National Osteoporosis Society Support Group

Try this and boogie

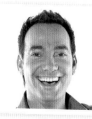

Try the 'Boogie for your Bones' Dance designed by Craig Revel Horwood, Patron of the National Osteoporosis Society. It's great fun: *www.nos.org.uk*

Help us celebrate a decade of our Breast Cancer Care Ben Nevis Challenge

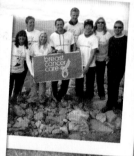

breast
cancer
care

Imagine standing at the top of magnificent Ben Nevis looking across the beautiful Western Highlands. An amazing achievement, made all the more special knowing your support will have helped so many people affected by breast cancer.

26–28 September 2014

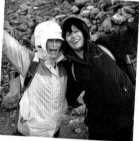

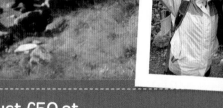

Register today for just £50 at
www.breastcancercare.org.uk/ben-nevis-challenge

- Two night's accommodation
- Return coach transfers from Glasgow
- All meals
- Qualified guides on the mountain

- Exclusive Ben Nevis T-shirt
- Fundraising and training support
- Celebration evening and certificate
- Amazing memories

Quote code BNC14

Get into...
fitness classes

A variety of gym work and classes can help develop fitness, strength and flexibility

Wt's important to find something that works for you and suits your lifestyle and pocket. The options are endless. You can join a private gym, pay-as-you-go at your local leisure centre or find a friendly class in your local village hall.

Mix things up to avoid boredom, so include a variety of gym work and classes to focus on all aspects of fitness, strength and flexibility.

Stay on track

Having a commitment to a class at a set time, especially if you've pre-booked, is a great way to keep you motivated.

Social scene

The social interaction from meeting people and friends at the gym or in your class is important, especially if you're retired or on your own.

TOP 5 CLASSES

❶ Spinning Group cycling classes to music. Boost your cardiovascular fitness and leg strength.

❷ Circuit training A mix of cardiovascular and strength exercises set out in a circuit format for all-round fitness training.

❸ TRX Using straps suspended from the ceiling, you use your own bodyweight as resistance to build strength, power and develop your core.

❹ Zumba The UK's hottest fitness craze combines a series of aerobic and dance moves to Latin music.

❺ Kettlebells Involves swinging a cannonball-shaped weight in a series of moves and lifts. Builds strength, fitness and core.

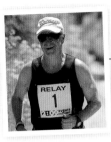

Bill's Story

Bill Bullen 74, is a regular gym user and shows it's never too late to start

"After my wife died in 2004, I found that going to the gym helped me meet people and got me fitter. I do four sessions a week of spinning, yoga and weight training, and do 60 press-ups a day. I joined a beginners' running club when I was 70. I've now done a few 10k races, half marathons and the South Downs Marathon relay. The social side of the gym and the running group is important to me and I've made some good friends. And I'm probably fitter than I ever have been."

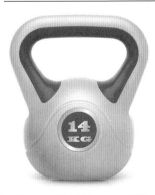

Get into...

pilates

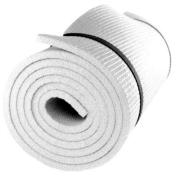

> " *If, at the age of 30, you're stiff and out of shape, you're old. If, at 60, you're supple and strong then you're young* "

Joseph Pilates

Far from being a current fitness craze, pilates was founded in the early 1920s as a form of rehabilitation by Joseph Pilates. Today, there's a wide variety of methods and techniques, and the focus is on wellbeing and posture. Fundamentally, pilates is a blend of strength and flexibility training, suitable for all ages and abilities, men and women. It's often recommended by physiotherapists and doctors as a treatment to help chronic back pain or postural and muscular imbalances. It works the core muscles around the spine, pelvis and shoulder girdle, and can help with injury rehabilitation and mobility.

Typically, pilates is a mat work class done on the floor. It can also be done on a reformer, or with a ball, ring or other pieces of equipment, which create additional resistance or support.

Benefits

The benefits of pilates are endless, and it can be tailored to your own needs and ability. While it's an excellent choice for older people due to the focus on balance, mobility, strength and flexibility, younger people and athletes also benefit from postural awareness and improved core stability:
www.pilatesfoundation.com

PILATES DVD

If you can't get to a class, try a home DVD such as Stott Pilates Express Series:
www.physicalcompany.co.uk

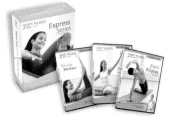

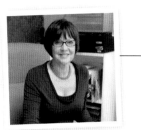

Sandra's Story

Sandra Bates, 64, does three pilates classes a week

"I've always enjoyed exercise and fitness classes, but as I got older I was getting more injuries and needed to do something different. Pilates keeps me strong and more mobile, and I love the social side of the classes. My core is stronger, my posture is better and I can pick things up off the floor and move more easily. It's helped my shoulder injury, too. I can't think of anything else I'd rather do. We need to look after ourselves as we get older, and pilates is the way I do that." *With thanks to www.studioonepilates.co.uk*

Getting the best from a
home gym

Who needs the gym anyway? Invest in a few pieces of equipment and you have everything you need for a great resistance workout at home. Rethink the way you exercise. Short workouts of 15-20 minutes are easy to squeeze into your day and more effective. Find achievable and realistic ways to make it work for you

❶ SUSPENSION TRAINER

Hang the trainer from the ceiling and use your body weight for a great core and strength workout.

❷ HAND WEIGHTS

For a variety of arm, shoulder and upper body toning. You may want a few different weights.

❸ YOGA MAT

A good mat for floor work is essential. Choose a yoga-style sticky mat that doesn't slip around.

❹ DYNABANDS

The orginal home exercise resistance tool. Use for all manner of exercises and corrective postural work.

❺ PILATES DVD

A great alternative if you can't get to an actual class. Stott Pilates Express Series 30-minute workouts is ideal.

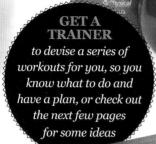

GET A TRAINER *to devise a series of workouts for you, so you know what to do and have a plan, or check out the next few pages for some ideas*

6 FOAM ROLLER
A form of self myofascial release or massage to improve flexibility, function, performance and reduce injuries.

7 BOSU
Doing exercises on an unstable platform makes your core work harder and is great for balance.

8 STEP
Choose one that has adjustable heights. Use for step-ups, as a bench and for a wide range of strength work.

9 KETTLE BELL
Incorporate some swings and kettle bell moves into your workout. Get a trainer to check your technique.

10 FIT BALL
For a range of core exercises, wall squats or even sitting at your desk. Choose the right size for you.

Mobility
training

*Some gentle, daily mobility exercises can help you move
more freely – and make you feel fantastic!*

Most of us lack movement through the spine and pelvis, which can create problems in other areas of the body, leaving us feeling stiff and immobile. Lack of mobility can also compromise our movement when we run, walk, swim or cycle, affecting performance.

These movements are aimed at increasing mobility rather than stretching the muscles, and will help you move more freely. Plus, they make you feel great!

Slot these exercises into your day whenever you can – some can be done sitting at your desk – or put them together for a specific mobility session. Try to do some mobility exercises each day and work on the areas you feel most restricted.

These exercises are generally very gentle, safe and suitable for everyone.

NOTE If you have a health condition, please check with your doctor or physiotherapist before doing these exercises. If you feel any discomfort or pain, stop immediately and consult a medical professional for advice.

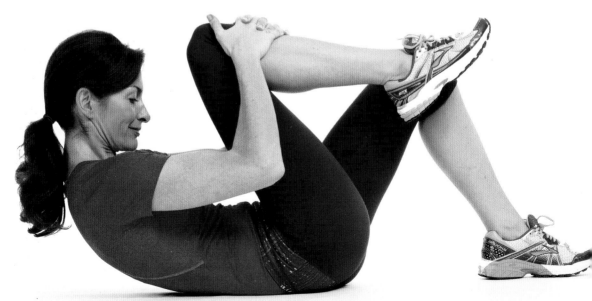

Knee rolls
20-30 repetitions

Increases mobility through the lumbar and thoracic spine and pelvis.

1 Lie on your back, knees bent and arms out to the side.

2 Keeping your shoulders on the floor and your feet together, let your knees roll from one side to the other in a gentle, fluid movement. Allow your foot to lift up, but keep your hips planted.

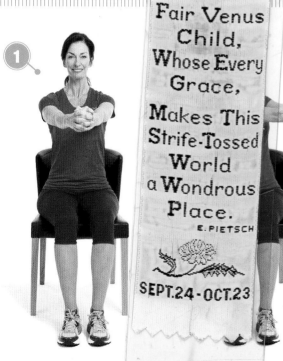

LIBRA

Fair Venus
Child,
Whose Every
Grace,
Makes This
Strife-Tossed
World
a Wondrous
Place.
E. PIETSCH

SEPT.24 - OCT.23

Shoulder rotations
20-30 repetitions

Helps to increase mobility through the mid-back (thoracic) area. A great one to do at your desk if you're feeling a bit stiff.

1 Sit on a table or chair with your knees at 90 degrees. Avoid having your back supported. Clasp your hands out in front of you with your arms straight at chest height.

2 Keeping your hips facing forwards and your shoulders relaxed, swing your arms in a slow pendulum movement from side to side. Let your head follow your arms, but keep your pelvis pointing to the front.

MOBILITY EXERCISES

Side slides
20-30 repetitions

A lovely release for your thoracic spine and muscles in the mid back.

1 Sit on your chair with your knees at 90 degrees, hips facing the front, and your arms out to the sides at shoulder height.

2 Aim to lift and slide your ribs over your pelvis from side to side in a flowing glide movement.

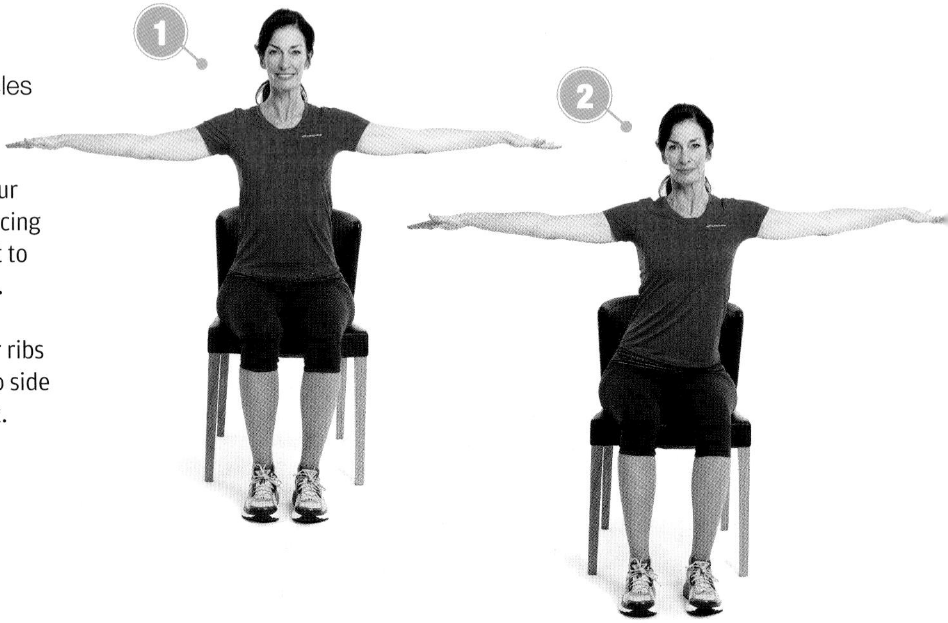

FLATTENED

ARCHED

Pelvic tilts
Try 8-10 repetitions x 2 sets twice per day

Increases movement through the pelvis.

1 Lie on your back, knees bent, arms down by your side. Keep your chest and shoulders still and relaxed.

2 Simply arch and flatten your lower back, aiming to get some movement through the pelvis. Don't over exaggerate the movement. Aim for a slow, fluid, rocking motion.

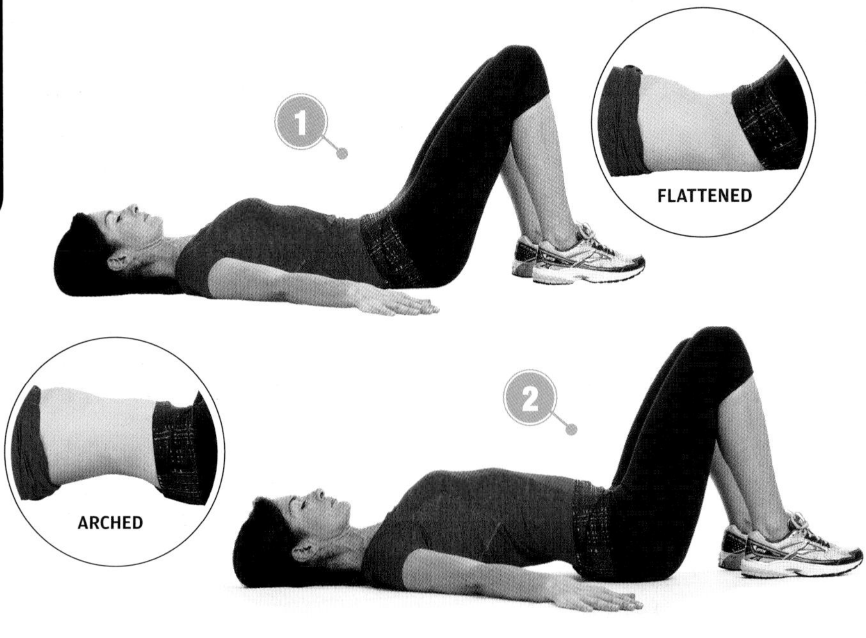

Alternate knee to chest
**8-10 repetitions x 2 sets
(build up to 15 x 4 sets)**

Helps to create movement through the spine and improve lower back flexion.

1 Lie on your back, knees bent. Lift your head and chest off the floor, and tuck your chin into your chest.

2 Lift one knee towards your chest and lift your chin towards your knee. Repeat on the other leg. Keep the movement fluid and gentle. This is not an abdominal exercise.

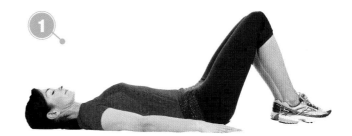

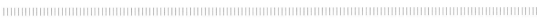

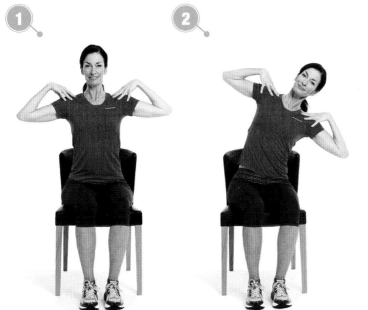

Side bends
**8-10 repetitions x 2 sets
(build up to 15 x 4 sets)**

Improves movement at the waist and in the lumbar spine.

1 Sit on your chair, feet flat on the floor. Put your hands on your shoulders, with elbows out to the sides.

2 Keeping your hips still, bend down from side to side, aiming your elbow to your hip.

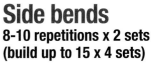

MOBILITY EXERCISES

Self Myofascial Release

This is a great way to release the fascia within the muscle and is similar to getting a sports massage. It helps to break down any scar tissue and allows the body to move more freely. It's very popular with athletes and recreational exercisers of all abilities. Highly recommended for everyone.

❯ Work your way slowly up the muscle, adjusting your body position as you go. Stop on any hot spots. Make sure you breathe and relax. It can be a bit eye watering at first! Aim for three full rolls up each muscle.

Note: Don't foam roll if you have high blood pressure, and avoid rolling over varicose veins. Check with your doctor if you're unsure if it's suitable for you.

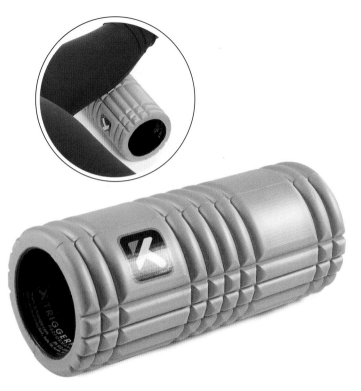

Quad rolling
A total of 9 full, slow rolls

❯ Lying face down, position the roller at the bottom of your thigh, near your knee.

❯ Balance your weight over your arms and position your other knee bent out to the side. Slowly roll up towards your hip.

❯ Repeat three times. Adjust your position so you can roll the outside edge of the quad, the main body of the muscle and the inner edge.

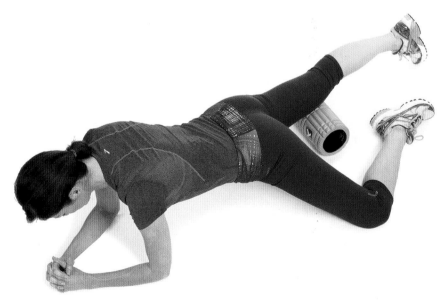

Calf rolling

Complete 3 full rolls up the middle, outer and inner sections of the muscle

▶ Position the roller at the bottom of your calf muscle and take your weight onto your hands.

▶ Slowly roll up your calf, stopping on hot spots and adjusting your weight and hand position as you go.

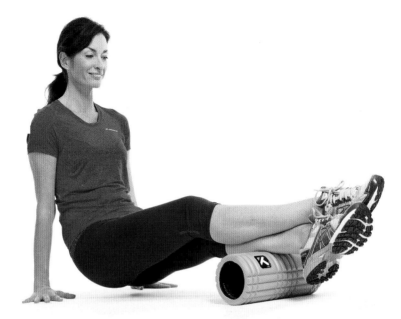

MOBILITY EXERCISES

TIP

Avoid areas of bone and focus on soft tissue. Adjust your weight as you go

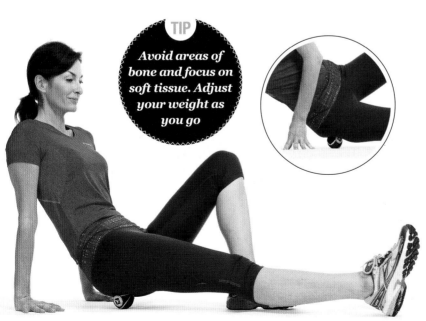

Glute ball release

▶ Lie or sit on the Trigger Point Ball under your glute (buttock) muscle. Move it gently around. When you find a hot spot, stop and breathe, allowing the muscle to relax.

▶ Adjust your weight on the ball to achieve the desired pressure.

▶ Try to work through all areas of the glutes and hip.

Strength training

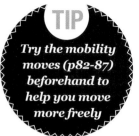

TIP

Try the mobility moves (p82-87) beforehand to help you move more freely

Strength training helps prevent loss of bone mass, builds muscle and improves your balance

Resistance training is one of the most important things you can do as you get older. Maintaining muscle mass can offset some of the effects of ageing, such as sarcopenia, osteoporosis and fat gain, and should be the focus of your fitness programme. Staying strong will also improve your sport performance, especially if you're a runner or cyclist, and may help to prevent injury.

We're not talking about heavy weight training or spending hours in the gym. The focus here is on using a range of light resistance and body weight exercises to build and maintain a strong, resilient body. The key is to incorporate sessions regularly and consistently and for shorter bursts rather than lengthy workouts.

You can slot some of these exercises into your day (squats while waiting for the kettle to boil) or combine them to make up a circuit-style workout, which should take around 20 minutes. This combination of exercises will give you a great all-round workout.

NOTE As with all exercise programmes, speak to your doctor before starting. If you feel any pain or discomfort at any time when exercising, stop and consult a medical professional.

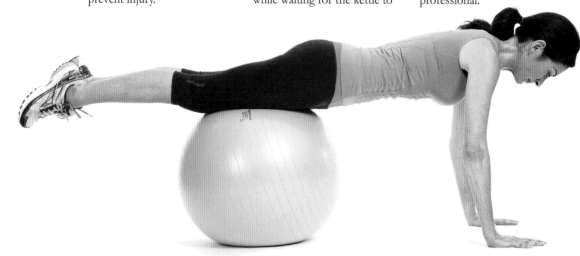

TVA brace
3-5 repetitions

Being more aware of your Transverse Abdominals (TVA) is important for core strength and pelvis control.

1 Lie on your back with your knees bent. Place your fingers on your stomach, about an inch in from your hip bones. Without pushing your back into the floor, try to brace your TVA without moving any other part of your body. You should feel the muscles contract under your fingers. Hold for 15 seconds then release. Repeat, holding for up to 30 seconds, then repeat three to five times.

2 Progression: while holding the brace position, lift your heel one inch off the ground, pause, then lower and repeat on the other leg. Avoid any movement in the pelvis. Repeat 10 times very slowly.

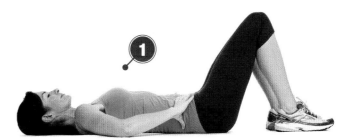

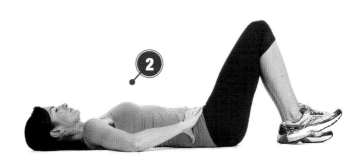

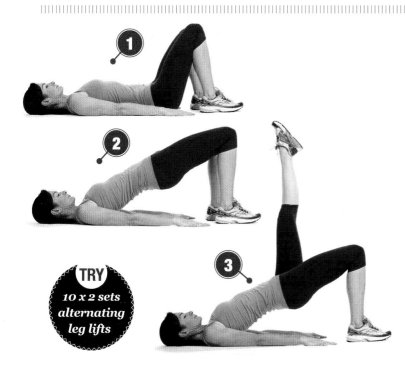

TRY
10 x 2 sets alternating leg lifts

Glute bridge
Sets: hold for 30 seconds; build up to 60 seconds x 3 sets

Strengthening your glute (buttock) muscles will help with posture and prevent back problems.

1 Lie on your back, knees bent, arms by your side. Keep shoulders relaxed.

2 Push your hips up into a bridge position. Squeeze your glutes and hold for 30 seconds. Slowly lower and repeat. Build up to holding for 60 seconds and repeat three times.

3 Progression: in your bridge position, try lifting your foot and straighten your leg. Your pelvis shouldn't move.

Side plank with leg raises

8-10 repetitions x 2-3 sets on each side

This is a combo move working your obliques on the side of your waist and your all-important glutes.

1 Lie on your side with your knee bent and top leg straight. Push up into a side plank position with your elbow under your shoulder. Hold the position using your side abdominal muscles.

2 Lift your arm up to the ceiling. Lift your top leg as high as you can and lower. Repeat the leg lift movement. You should feel it in the side of your hip and glutes.

TIP
A great exercise for runners

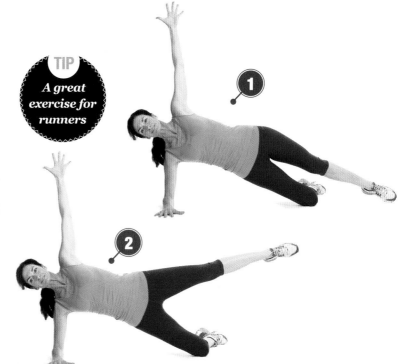

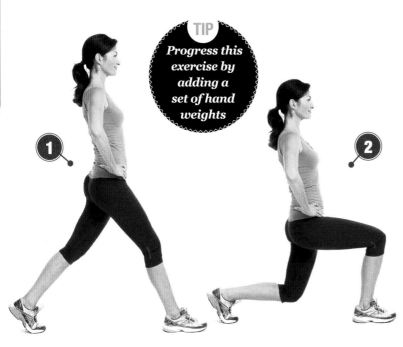

TIP
Progress this exercise by adding a set of hand weights

Basic lunge

10-15 repetitions on each leg x 2-3 sets

One of the best exercises for your legs and glutes.

1 Start in a split stance position. Both legs straight, up on your back toe, hips facing forwards.

2 Then lunge, bending both knees and dropping your bodyweight centrally between both feet. Aim to get both knees to around 90 degrees. The back knee drops to the floor. Keep chest lifted and hips tucked under. Push back up to straight leg position and repeat.

Single arm rows with dynaband

**Repeat 15-20 times
x 3 sets on each arm**

This works arm and shoulders in a fluid movement.

1 Sit or stand holding one end of a dynaband with your arm straight. The other end should be attached to a solid object (door handle or hook) so that the band is around chest height.

2 Keeping your chest and pelvis facing forwards, pull the band backwards until your hand is by your ribs. Keep your shoulder down and wrist straight. Adjust your position to get the right resistance.

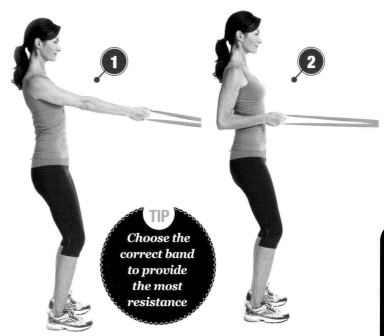

TIP

Choose the correct band to provide the most resistance

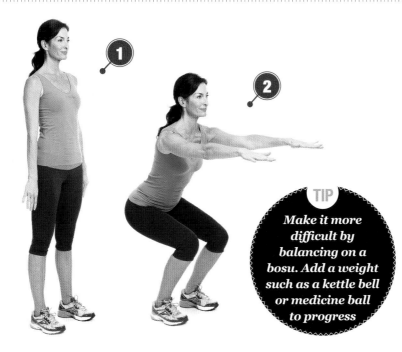

TIP

Make it more difficult by balancing on a bosu. Add a weight such as a kettle bell or medicine ball to progress

Simple squats

**10-15 repetitions
x 2-3 sets**

A classic but very effective move for your legs and glutes.

1 Stand with feet hip distance apart and drop your weight onto your heels.

2 Arms out in front of you, squat down, engaging your glute muscles. Avoid arching your back. Squat as low as you comfortably can, then drive back up to standing.

STRENGTH EXERCISES

Hamstring ball rolls

10-15 reps x 2-3 sets

Specifically targets the hamstrings and glutes.

1 Lie on your back with your calves on the ball and arms by your sides.

2 Lift your hips up to a bridge position, keeping shoulders relaxed. Keep your hips up, pull the ball towards you using your feet. Roll back out again and repeat the hamstring curl movement, maintaining high hips at all times.

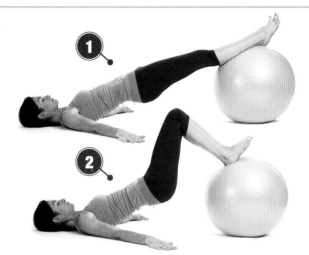

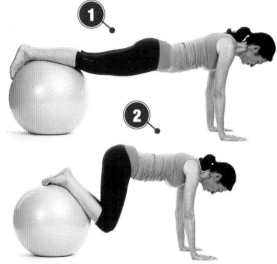

Knee pulls

10-15 reps x 2-3 sets

1 In a press-up position with your hands under your shoulders, put your feet on the ball. Get your balance on the ball and use your abdominals to hold your position.

2 Slowly pull the ball towards you, curling your knees to your chest, then push it back out again in a fluid movement. Keep your hips in alignment. Keep your shoulders strong and focus on using your stomach, back and glutes.

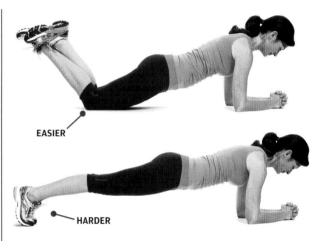

EASIER

HARDER

Classic plank

Hold for 20 seconds then lower. Repeat 2-3 times. Build up to holding for 60 seconds

➤ Start with elbows under your shoulders and forearms on the floor. Push up into a straight plank position, either on your toes (harder) or on your knees (easier).

➤ Get your body in alignment from your head all the way through your hips and knees. Avoid sagging your lower back or arching too high. Maintain a strong position without moving or shaking.

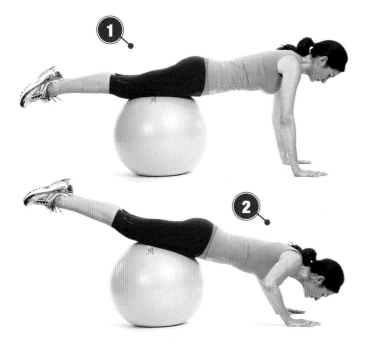

Ball press-up

Aim for 10 reps and build up to 15 x 3 sets

Press-ups off the fitball are easily adapted to your own ability. Having the ball closer to your feet makes it harder.

1 Legs on the ball - anywhere between your hips and feet, depending on your ability.

2 With your hands directly under your shoulders, take your nose towards the floor, then push up in a strong and fluid movement, keeping your body in a straight line.

Upright row squat with kettle bell

Repeat 10-15 reps x 2-3 sets

A great combo move for an all-over workout.

1 Squat with your toes pointing out slightly. Avoid arching your lower back; keep it strong. Hold the kettle bell with both hands and let it hang between your legs.

2 In one fluid movement, drive up with the legs and pull up with your arms, leading with your elbows and keeping the kettle bell at chest height. Squat back down again, lowering the bell at the same time and keeping your weight in your heels.

TIP
Most women will start with a 4-6kg kettlebell and men 10-14kg

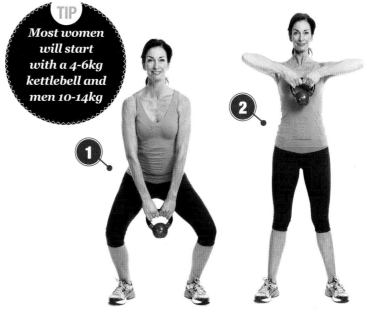

STRENGTH EXERCISES

Fitness round-up

Contrary to popular belief, running doesn't cause arthritis. The US National Runners' Health Study published data that showed runners are actually half as likely to develop osteoarthritis or to need a hip or knee replacement compared to walkers.

MAKING A CONSCIOUS CHOICE to improve your quality of life through health and fitness is the first step. But don't rely on willpower or just hoping it will happen. You have to take control and make it work for you.

We're talking about exercise, the sort of exercise that raises your heart rate and gets you breathless. The sort that keeps your muscles strong and flexible, and your body toned. And the sort that will help you to stay active, mobile and healthy well into your 70s, 80s and beyond.

While a stroll to the shops is a great way to stay active, it's probably not enough to offset the effects of ageing or make much difference to your cardiovascular function or muscle mass.

25% ▶ of people gain weight once they've joined the gym, as they give themselves treats after a workout. Try to view the reward in the healthy lifestyle changes you've made instead of a "gift" for yourself after exercising. Feeling fitter, sleeping better, laughing more – these are the rewards.

Awareness is key, so find out exactly how active you are (or not) by wearing a pedometer, such as a Fitbug: *www.fitbug.com*. It can be a big wake-up call, as most people significantly overestimate their activity level.

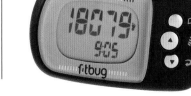

Recent research found that physical activity may be as effective as medication in managing some long-term conditions such as heart disease, stroke and pre-diabetes.

FINAL WORD
We may not be able to prevent the inevitable physiological changes related to ageing, but there's a lot we can do to slow them down and stay as fit, healthy and strong as possible.

'*Let food be thy medicine, thy medicine shall be thy food*'

Hippocrates

Nutrition priorities

We have an abundance of nutritional information at our fingertips. Advice can be found online, in books and magazines, but it can be conflicting and overwhelming, often leaving us confused about our diet and the choices we should make

Expert opinion also seems to change rapidly: is high fat and low carb better, or should we eat low fat and high protein? And what exactly does that mean for our day to day lives?

There's no doubt, however, that our diet plays a very important role in our health and prevention of disease, not to mention providing optimum fuel for activity. The World Cancer Research Fund estimates that around 38% of all cancers could be avoided through lifestyle changes, so eating a healthy diet has never been more important.

As we age, our nutritional requirements change too, and we must make sure we eat the right foods of the best, freshest quality if we can – and reduce our intake of processed food. Our metabolism naturally drops as we age; we lose muscle mass and may become more sedentary, so we need fewer calories. If we don't change our diet or our activity levels; or both, we can easily put on weight.

Over the next few pages, we'll take a look at some of the more important nutritional concerns for older people including vitamin D, calcium, vitamin C, magnesium, fibre, protein and iron as well as showing you how to achieve a balanced diet.

We hope to dispel some nutrition myths and provide up-to-date advice, top tips, expert comments and recipes.

Eating a healthy diet is vital for our wellbeing and prevention of disease. But we don't just eat for health. Food is an important aspect of social interaction and pleasure too. So keep things in perspective and aim for a sensible balance.

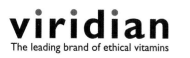

The leading brand of ethical vitamins

Care for others as you care for yourself

65+ Multi

Specially formulated with age-appropriate vitamins, minerals, digestive enzymes and energy factors for the over 65s.

PURITY · CHARITY · ENVIRONMENT
For your nearest specialist health store visit www.viridian-nutrition.com

viridian

ENHANCED ABSORPTION

65+ MULTI

With Co-Q10, B12 & ALA

60 VEGETARIAN CAPSULES

PURCHASE · THANK YOU · CHARITY DONATION

This formula has been cross-checked for safety with the most common age-related prescribed medications.
Check with your GP if you are currently taking prescription medicines.

Balancing
your diet

Eating a wide range of foods, especially "real foods",
is vital for our health and wellbeing

No one single food on its own contains all the essential nutrients that the human body needs for good health, which is why it's so important to eat a balanced diet. Eating a wide range of foods from the various different food groups is most likely the best way to provide the correct nutrients we need, and vital for our health and wellbeing.

But what exactly is a balanced diet and how do we put it into practice?

Current national guidelines in the UK recommend that we base our diet on the Eatwell Plate (see overleaf). A diet based on the correct balance of foods from all the sections – starchy foods such as potatoes, rice and pasta; with plenty of fruit and vegetables; some protein-rich foods such as meat, fish and pulses; milk and dairy foods; and limited amounts of processed and sugary foods – should provide all the nutrients you need. This illustrates how faddy diets, which eliminate entire food groups, can be very unhealthy.

Powerful protein

As you age, it's essential to give more consideration to your protein intake. It's thought that people over the age of 50 may require more protein in their diet, so try to include some protein at every meal. Foods such as meat, pulses, dairy produce, fish, nuts, eggs, and vegetarian products such as quorn and tofu are all good sources of protein. Protein is essential for muscle repair, recovery after exercise and has been linked to the prevention of muscle loss in older people. It also helps to stabilise your appetite and blood sugar levels, meaning that you'll have fewer cravings and feel less hungry.

Putting it into practice

But eating healthily doesn't have to be complicated. In very simple terms, aim to keep your consumption of processed food to a minimum. This means eating "real foods" close

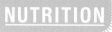
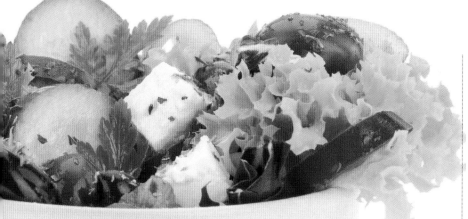

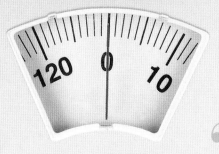

> *Try to include a balance of protein, fat and carbohydrate in every meal and snack*

5 TOP TIPS TO ACHIEVE A BALANCED DIET

1 Try to include a balance of protein, fat and carbohydrate in every meal and snack. Choose a high-protein breakfast of eggs, or include nuts and seeds to stabilise your appetite.

2 Avoid demonising a food or food group by labeling it bad or naughty. Every food has a place, and it's the balance that counts.

3 Portion sizes of meat and fish should be around the size of a deck of cards or the palm of your hand.

4 Don't be scared of fat, but try to get it from "real" sources – meat, fish, nuts, dairy, oils and so on – rather than processed foods.

5 Portions of carbohydrate – pasta, rice, bread, potatoes and so on – should be the size of your fist. Carbs are easy to overeat, so make sure your portion size doesn't creep up.

DITCH THE DIET

"There are many faddy diets on the market, and these tend to restrict certain foods groups, depriving our body of essential vitamins, minerals and macronutrients, which are required for our overall health," explains Nutritional Therapist Emily Whitehead from BetterYou.

"Restricting food groups may also lead to nutritional deficiencies, cravings, hunger and food binges. Faddy diets may help you to lose weight at the beginning, but they're unsustainable in the long term, and the majority of dieters put the weight straight back on after they've finished dieting."

The eatwell plate

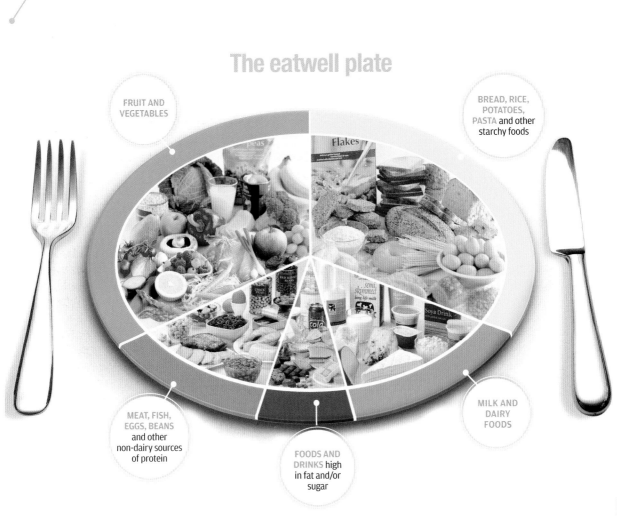

FRUIT AND VEGETABLES

BREAD, RICE, POTATOES, PASTA and other starchy foods

Flakes

MEAT, FISH, EGGS, BEANS and other non-dairy sources of protein

FOODS AND DRINKS high in fat and/or sugar

MILK AND DAIRY FOODS

Use the eatwell plate to help you get the balance right. It shows how much you should eat from each food group

to their natural state, and reducing your consumption of cakes, biscuits, ready meals, refined pasta and bread, takeaways, processed snacks, soft drinks and sugary foods.

"The ultimate message is the same and really quite simple," explains Martin McDonald, Director of the

nutrition consultancy www. Mac-Nutrition.com and Nutritional Advisor for Total. "Just eat real food. That way, it's almost impossible to over-consume processed carbs, and the fat you do eat will come from natural sources. If you eat 'real food' and avoid processed junk,

you're likely to start self-regulating your appetite and you'll achieve a more balanced diet without over-thinking it. Sugar cravings will lessen and your blood sugar levels will stabilise. With my clients, the first three things I teach them to support the 'real food message' are eat more

PUBLIC HEALTH ENGLAND IN ASSOCIATION WITH THE WELSH AND SCOTTISH GOVERNMENT AND THE FOOD STANDARDS AGENCY IN NORTHERN IRELAND

vegetables, consume protein with each meal and become a conscientious eater in terms of portion sizes."

"Healthy" isn't always healthy

Quite often the foods that are sold to us as healthy options are quite literally the opposite. "An excellent example of this is yoghurt," continues Martin MacDonald. "It's far healthier to eat something like a natural Greek yoghurt, which is naturally higher in protein and fat than a diet yoghurt that's low in fat and loaded with sugar or artificial sweeteners but is promoted as being 'healthy'. Read the labels carefully. Food companies can use terms like organic, gluten free and low in fat or salt to make an otherwise unhealthy product seem like it's a good choice. In general, good, "natural" food will not have to make health claims."

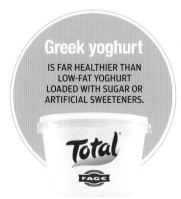

Greek yoghurt

IS FAR HEALTHIER THAN LOW-FAT YOGHURT LOADED WITH SUGAR OR ARTIFICIAL SWEETENERS.

Total

FAGE

ANTI-AGEING NUTRITION TIPS

Anti-ageing nutrition tips from Nutritionist Miguel Toribio-Mateus

"As you age, keeping your body in top condition is akin to keeping a classic car. You wouldn't let it rust just because it's not a new model. In fact, you'd make an extra effort to find the right parts and to take it to a specialist garage, where it can get the expert, high- quality service it deserves. The same goes with your body. Treat it with the respect and care it deserves by leading a healthy lifestyle and eating a diet rich in fish, green veg, fibre from fruit, whole grains and pulses.

When out shopping, load your trolley with deep green vegetables to boost your calcium and magnesium intake. Magnesium supports energy and cardiovascular health, and calcium is essential for bones. Also try a daily handful of walnuts, and oily fish three times a week to help keep your joints supple and pain free. My favourites are salmon, mackerel and sardines.

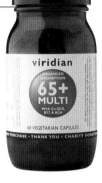
FUEL AFTER EXERCISE

Nutrition really comes into its own after exercise. Eat the right thing immediately after a hard training session, and you'll recover faster and reduce risk of injury.

After exercise, you have a window of about one hour where your muscles are most receptive to being restocked with glycogen. Use this time to refuel with a snack combining a 3:1 ratio of carbs to protein. Research suggests a glass of milk provides the right balance of nutrients and helps you recover faster. A US study even shows low-fat chocolate milk as a better post-workout recovery drink than sports drinks – and shaves off more fat.

Eating habits
& weight management

Diets don't work... at least not in the long term. You may lose weight for a short period of time, but eventually the weight creeps on again and you're back to square one

According to life coach and weight loss guru Pete Cohen (*www. weightlossguru.com*),

"People go back to what they know. If you want to lose weight and keep it off, there's a lot more to it than what you eat. Don't do what everyone else is doing, or follow the current trendy diet; work out your own path and find a system that works for you."

So if diets don't work, how do you lose weight?

There are literally hundreds of reasons why people get overweight. And those reasons are different for all of us.

"You might eat when you're stressed, bored or depressed," explains Pete. "You might not be very active, you might eat too much of a particular type of food, eat too fast, or your stress levels might be so high you inhibit your ability to burn fat. Or it may be all of those things. You need to work out why you're overweight and what you can do about it."

Action steps

1 Try a little soul searching. How do I feel about my weight? What's got me to this point? What are the triggers that cause me to eat? Be honest with yourself.

2 Then imagine the consequences of doing nothing. Picture yourself in 10 years' time... really visualise what you might look like and how that will affect your mobility, lifestyle and health. Then do the opposite – picture yourself fit, healthy, mobile and with an active lifestyle. Which image do you like most?

3 A food diary can be a powerful tool to raise awareness and pick up patterns about your eating and emotions. Don't just write down what you eat, but record why you're eating (bored, stressed, hungry – are you really hungry?) and your feelings at the time. Then look for patterns and triggers, and

It won't be easy, so be prepared and work out what you need to make it work

❯ You need to take personal responsibility – hold yourself accountable. The only person who can do this is you.

❯ Write down what you're going to do – get it scheduled. Get it done. Don't feel overwhelmed.

❯ Focus on the actions not the outcome. Instead of a "lose 10lb by Christmas" goal, target the small changes that will get you there.

❯ You need support, so get a buddy. Online groups work well where you can support and encourage each other. *www.weightlossguru.com*

work out what you can do to change.

4 Then make a list. What are your reasons for losing weight? You need reasons to make it real. Make a list and think carefully about what it is you want and why. The longer your list, the more compelling it will be.

5 Then work out the best course of action. "I encourage people not to do too many things at once," says Pete, "but just to change two or three things. Stick to it, master it and then move on. Focus on positive 'I can do' steps rather than negative 'I must stop' changes."

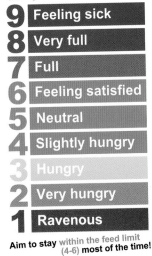

Hunger-Fullness Scale

Use this scale to rate your hunger just before you eat & your fullness when you stop eating!

9 **Feeling sick**
8 **Very full**
7 **Full**
6 **Feeling satisfied**
5 **Neutral**
4 **Slightly hungry**
3 **Hungry**
2 **Very hungry**
1 **Ravenous**

Aim to stay within the feed limit (4-6) most of the time!

Are you really hungry?

Get in tune with your hunger and satiety by using a hunger scale.

Your changing
nutritional
needs

Getting the right nutrients and vitamins as your body's requirements change is crucial, so let's take a look at what you need...

As we get older, our bodies, and our nutritional needs, begin to change. We need to make sure we're getting the right nutrients and in the correct amounts. 'Age specific' nutrients include Vitamin D, Calcium, Vitamin B12, Iron and Magnesium.

If your eating habits change; you eat less or snack more, your body may not get the right balance of these essential nutrients. You may need to consider supplements or fortified foods. Get advice from your GP or a registered dietician. See www.bda.org.

In the presence of sunlight, our skin can produce the vitamin D we need, but 70-80% of the population may be deficient in this important vitamin. B12 is a vital vitamin as we get older, too

Vitamin D

Known as the sunshine vitamin, it important for overall health, immunity and healthy bones, and one of the most topical vitamins in nutrition and health at the moment. It's also important to aid calcium absorption. We get very little vitamin D from food, but our body makes it when we have exposure to sunlight.

A lack of vitamin D has been linked to Alzheimer's, diabetes, cancer, asthma, high blood pressure, depression and SAD. Signs of deficiency are vague, but may include tiredness, general aches and pains, and depression.

Experts estimate that 70-80% of the population may be deficient in vitamin D. If you're housebound, don't spend much time outside or are over the age of 70, you may be more at risk. If you think you might be deficient or at risk, ask your GP for a blood test to check your vitamin D levels. More information at *www.vitamindcouncil.org*.

Vitamin D is a fat-soluble vitamin, and found mainly in oily fish and some fortified cereals. It's unlikely you'll meet your vitamin D needs through diet alone. Try DLux oral spray by *www.betteryou.uk.com* and aim to get outside in the sunlight as much as possible.

Vitamin B12

B12 is found in animal foods such as meat, eggs, milk, fish and poultry, as well as fortified cereals. It's important for maintenance of a healthy nervous system function, and vital for memory, cognitive function and other neurological processes.

Even though a deficiency is rare, it's thought that our ability to absorb vitamin B12 may be impaired as we get older due to a decrease in the production of stomach acid. Vegetarians may struggle to get enough in their diet and could require a supplement.

Breakthrough research from the University of Oxford published in October 2013 suggested that B12 supplementation may reduce the rate of brain shrinkage, a symptom associated with memory loss and dementia, by 53%. This could turn out to be a significant finding for the future treatment of Alzheimer's. Try Vitamin B12 oral spray from *www.betteryou.uk.com.*

Consult your doctor, dietitian or a medical professional before taking vitamin supplements.

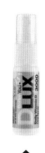

TRY DLUX
An optimal dosage of vitamin D delivered in every spray

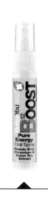

VITAMIN B12 ORAL SPRAY
Your natural daily requirement of vitamin B12 delivered easily and orally

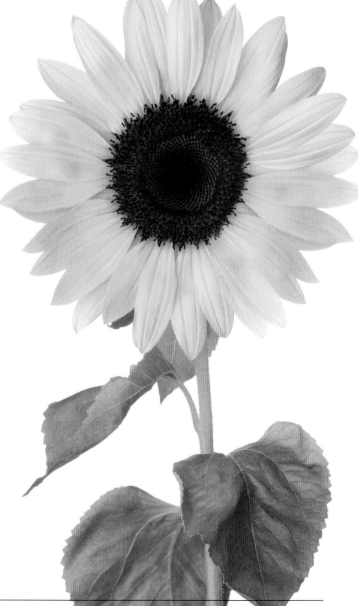

> *Vitamin D, known as the sunshine vitamin, is important for overall health*

Calcium

Reports suggest women with high calcium levels are at twice the risk of dying from heart disease, so it's important to get your facts on calcium straight

C alcium is the most abundant mineral in your body and vital not only for strong bones and teeth, but for several critical functions including vascular contraction, muscle function, nerve transmission, and hormonal secretion.

If you don't get enough calcium you can risk health problems related to weak bones. Bone loss can affect people over 50, especially post-menopausal women, where bone is lost more quickly than it's formed, increasing the risk of osteoporosis (see p28).

How much calcium do I need?

The amount needed in your diet varies throughout life, with a daily requirement of about 1000mg for men and women over 50 years, says Dr Nitu Bajekal, Consultant Gynaecologist, Spire Bushey Hospital (www.nitubajekal. co.uk). Post-menopausal women may require more – around 1,200mg daily.

If your diet is healthy and you exercise regularly, including strength exercises, Dr Bajekal recommends a daily multivitamin containing 200mg of calcium as well as vitamin D should be enough to protect your bones.

In addition to including calcium in your diet, protect yourself against osteopenia and osteoporosis, by exercising for 20-30 minutes a day and include muscle strengthening exercises.

Our expert says:

"Calcium can be found in a range of foods, and for many people, dairy products are an easy way to include calcium in the diet. Dark green leafy veg are also good sources, and almonds, sesame seeds and figs are also rich in calcium. Some products like tofu and some breakfast cereals are fortified with calcium." Sarah Leyland, National Osteoporosis Society.

Magnesium

Up to 75% of us may not get enough magnesium in our diet, which is required by every organ in the body

Magnesium is an important, and often overlooked, essential mineral required by every organ in the body. It's required for muscle and nerve function, needed for energy and maintains bone structure, regulating calcium balance.

Magnesium also calms the adrenal gland and helps to balance blood sugar. A study of 12,000 people over six years found that those with the lowest levels of magnesium had a 94% chance of developing diabetes.

Symptoms of low levels of magnesium include muscle spasms, tremors, cramps, twitching, and changes in blood pressure and heart rate.

Stress, raised cortisol levels, processed food, caffeine and alcohol can all lower your levels, and we also lose significant amounts through sweat loss. It's thought that 75% of us don't get enough magnesium in our diet.

Bone health

Magnesium encourages the body to absorb calcium, and is vital in the prevention and treatment of osteoporosis. It's thought we need both calcium and magnesium in conjunction with vitamin D for optimum bone health. The importance of magnesium isn't recent news. A study in 1990, in *The Journal of Reproductive Medicine*, found that magnesium supplementation, instead of calcium, increased bone density of post-menopausal women within one year. It's thought that magnesium may be more important for bone health than calcium.

Where is it found?

It's found in nuts, whole grains, dark green vegetables, fish and meat. Rich sources include pumpkin and sunflower seeds, bran, tofu, potatoes, baked beans and spinach. An easy way to include some magnesium in your diet is to snack on dried fruit and nut mixes or sprinkle wheatgerm on cereal.

Our expert says

"I see a lot of women who are worried about their calcium levels, especially around the menopause, but when tested the majority are low in magnesium."
Dr Marilyn Glenville,
www.marilynglenville.com

Magnesium oil spray

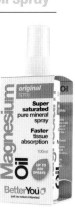

Magnesium Oil Spray from BetterYou delivers magnesium via the skin, entering cells immediately and replacing magnesium lost through sweat and stress. *www. betteryou.uk.com*

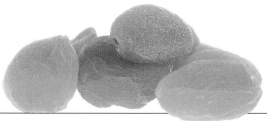

Iron

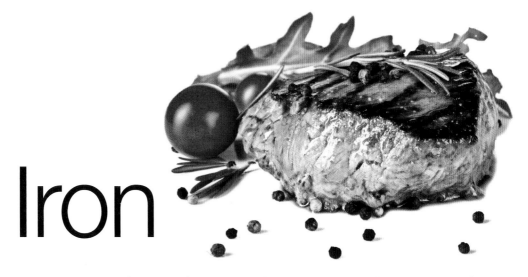

Iron is important for many functions in the body including formation of red blood cells and transport of oxygen to tissues. As you get older it is important to ensure an adequate iron intake and include iron rich foods in your diet

Good sources of Iron are meat and meat products, especially red meat and offal (such as liver and kidney); cereal products such as fortified breakfast cereals and bread; eggs; pulses such as baked beans and lentils; dried fruit, dark green vegetables such as curly kale and spinach.

Studies have found that iron intakes in older people are often significantly below the recommended level. It is thought this is due to possible changes in appetite, digestion difficulties and subsequent food choices.

In addition, iron absorption from the gut may also be

> **20% of people over the age of 65 diagnosed with anaemia are found to have an underlying condition**

reduced in older people and this coupled with low intakes, can increase the risk of iron deficiency anaemia.

Symptoms of anaemia include tiredness, lethargy and listlessness. Sometimes

in older people, anaemia can be the first symptom of an underlying gut disorder, so vital you get checked out by your GP if you have any symptoms. In fact around 20% of people over the age of 65 diagnosed with anaemia are found to have an underlying condition.

Good dietary consumption of iron along with foods providing vitamin C to aid absorption is vital. Good sources of Vitamin C include citrus fruits, kiwi fruit, tomatoes, potatoes and dark green vegetables. These foods should be eaten at the same time as the iron source for optimum absorption.

TREATING PROSTATE CANCER QUESTIONS & ANSWERS

For a **FREE** copy of this booklet please contact us at the address below.

This booklet has two aims:

- to help you become better informed about prostate cancer and its treatment.

- to guide you in the decisions you will make about your care with your doctor.

It cannot replace talking to your GP or hospital doctor.

If you can help us by raising funds for our research or to make a donation please contact us at the address below.

Your support is vital!

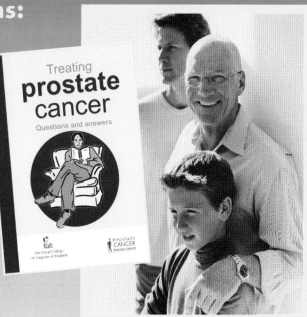

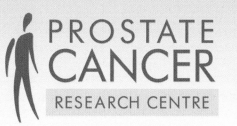

Prostate Cancer Research Centre • 67 Riding House Street • London • W1W 7EJ
Tel: 020 7679 9366 • email info@prostate-cancer-research.org.uk • www.prostate-cancer-research.org.uk

Your guide to super supplements

If you don't think you're getting sufficient vitamins and minerals from the foods you eat, there are a number of super supplements that will help boost you intake with ease. Here are our favourites

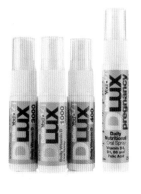

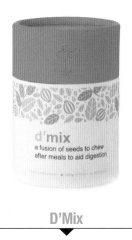

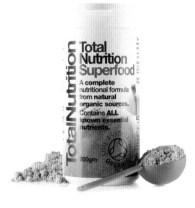

DLux

Vitamin D levels are a cause for concern as people spend more time indoors and SAD is on the increase. Only 10% of vitamin D comes from our diet, the rest from sunlight. A survey found that 90% of people in the UK could be vitamin D deficient. Boost your levels with the BetterYou DLux oral spray available in three strengths. *www.betteryou.uk.com*

D'Mix

As we age, our digestive system becomes more sluggish and slows down. D'Mix is a proprietary blend of eight herbs and spices to chew after meals, specially formulated to kick start the digestive process and to help bring your digestive system into its healthy, balanced state.
www.consciousfood.co.uk

Total Nutrition Superfood

Bursting with a powerful range of nutrients for optimum health, Total Nutrition Superfood provides nutritional support for every body system: skin, hair, nails, teeth, bones, digestive system and the immune system. 100% organic, raw food formula ensures the highest bio-availability and absorption.
www.betteryou.uk.com

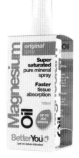

Magnesium Oil Spray

It's estimated that 75% of us don't get our daily requirement of magnesium from our diet. It's thought that absorption of magnesium via the skin is better than oral supplementation.
www.betteryou.uk.com

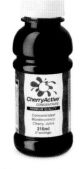

CherryActive

A serving of CherryActive has the same antioxidant content as eating 23 fruit and vegetables. Rich in anthocyanins, which possess natural anti-inflammatory properties, it may also help relieve arthritis.
www.cherryactive.co.uk

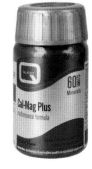

Cal-Mag Plus

Cal-Mag Plus multiminerals contain calcium, magnesium, and 11 essential minerals, including selenium, zinc and copper, to help prevent oxidative stress and promote a healthy immune system.
www.nutricentre.com

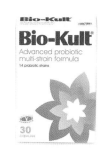

Bio-Kult probiotics

Probiotics help maintain a healthy digestive and immune system. Bio-Kult contains 14 strains of beneficial probiotic bacteria, proven to reach more areas of the gut, boosting vitamin B and D levels.
www.Bio-Kult.com

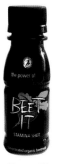

Beet IT

Beetroot juice is scientifically proven to lower blood pressure due to the high level of nitrates found in beetroot. It also increases endurance by around 15%. Take in a concentrated format.
www.beet-it.com

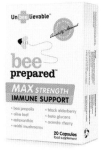

Bee Prepared

Bee propolis helps boost your immune system. Bee Prepared contains powerful antioxidants and bioflavonoid-rich nutrients with antiviral, antibacterial and antihistamine properties.
www.unbeelievable health.co.uk

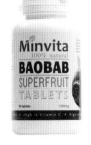

Baobab

From one of the oldest trees in the world, the Baobab fruit has two-and-a-half times more calcium than milk, and is high in fibre and vitamin C. In powdered form, it tastes great in smoothies and on cereals.
www.minvita.co.uk

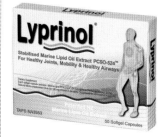

Lyprinol

Lyprinol is extracted from green-lipped mussel and contains a rare mix of marine lipid groups and unique omega 3 fatty acids. It's been shown to be 200-350 times more effective than standard fish oils.
www.lyprinol.co.uk

Fibre

This important nutrient isn't only about keeping our digestive systems running smoothly...

We all know that fibre is an essential part of a healthy diet, keeping our digestive system in working order, but it also helps to stabilise blood sugar and cholesterol levels – important in the management of diabetes and heart disease. In countries with traditionally high-fibre diets, diseases such as bowel cancer, diabetes and coronary heart disease are much less common than in Western countries. Most people in the UK don't get enough fibre in their diet.

Some of the potential outcomes that can occur if you don't eat enough fibre include constipation, irritable bowel syndrome (although sometimes a high intake of fibre can be worse for IBS), diverticular disease, heart disease and some cancers, including colon cancer.

There are two types of fibre, and we need to include both types in our diet:

Soluble fibre – Good sources of soluble fibre include fruits, vegetables, oat bran, barley, seed husks, flaxseed, psyllium, dried beans, lentils, peas, soy milk and soy products. Soluble fibre can also help with constipation and lower LDL cholesterol.

Insoluble fibre – Good sources include wheat bran, the skins of fruits and vegetables, nuts, seeds, dried beans and wholegrain foods. A major role of insoluble fibre is to add bulk and to prevent constipation and associated problems such as haemorrhoids.

Both types of fibre are beneficial to the body, and most plant foods contain a mixture of both types.

Important for older people

The digestive system slows down with age, so a high-fibre diet becomes even more important. Drinking plenty of fluid alongside a high-fibre diet is vital to prevent constipation and to aid digestion.

WAYS TO BOOST YOUR DAILY FIBRE INTAKE:

▶ Eat high-fibre breakfast cereals such as porridge.
▶ Switch to wholemeal or multigrain breads and brown rice.
▶ Add an extra vegetable to every evening meal.
▶ Snack on fruit, dried fruit, nuts or wholemeal crackers.
If you try to increase your intake, do it gradually to allow your body time to adapt. Increasing too quickly can lead to cramps, wind and bloating.

Claim your FREE copy of Saga Magazine today!

Have you enjoyed this Fit for Life MagBook? Want to know more about health, fitness and nutrition?

If so, we think you'll love Saga Magazine. Not only is it packed full of health news, tips and advice, it also covers homes, gardens, celebs, culture, recipes, royals, money, nostalgia, beauty, fashion and books.

But don't just take our word for it – claim your FREE issue today to find out what makes Saga Magazine the UK's bestselling monthly*.

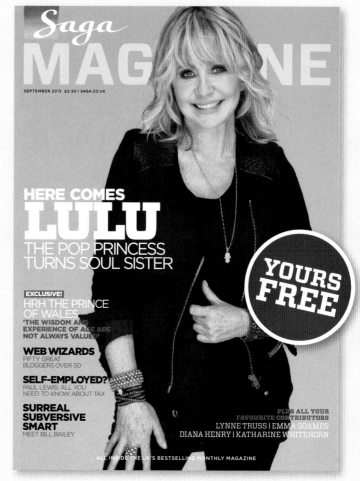

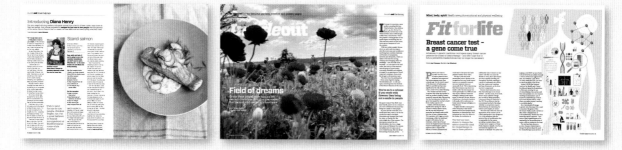

 Simply call **FREEPHONE 0800 056 1057** and quote the promotional code FIT14. Lines are open Monday to Friday, 9am-5pm.

Sugar

If you still think that eating fat is bad for you, think again. Experts are learning that it's the added sugar in food, which is actually driving the obesity epidemic, and the rise in diabetes and cardiovascular disease

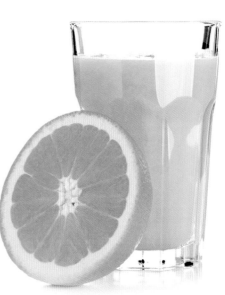

A recent article in the BMJ by Cardiologist Dr Aseem Malhotra, suggested that the consumption of sugar may have closer correlation to heart disease than dietary fat. And Dr Marilyn Glenville, author of 'Fat around the Middle' agrees that sugar is hugely damaging for our health.

Carbohydrates, especially wholegrains, however; are an important source of energy in our diet, especially for active people and shouldn't be avoided. It's the sugary, highly processed carbohydrate foods we need to be aware of. Limit your consumption of biscuits, cakes, sweets and sugary foods and drinks where possible and avoid processed 'low fat' foods, which are often loaded with sugar.

> 66 *One research study found a glass of orange juice contained more sugar than 3.5 doughnuts - more than a can of coke* 99

Dangerous Drinks

Watch out for seemingly 'healthy' choices such as orange juice and smoothies and don't be fooled by the marketing on the label promising health benefits. One research study found a glass of orange juice contained more sugar than 3.5 doughnuts – more than a can of coke. Sugar is sugar, regardless of the source.

Limit sugar in your diet

Sugar comes in many guises as glucose, fructose, lactose and sucrose in foods such as fruit, milk, honey, jam, syrup as well as processed foods, cakes and biscuits. They are all sources of sugar in our diet. Eating too much sugar causes insulin levels to rapidly rise and fall, putting strain on your metabolism, over time leading to heart disease, high blood pressure, arthritis and weight gain.

Try to maintain steady blood sugar levels by eating more protein and fat in your diet, avoiding the insulin spikes that come with eating sugary snacks and meals. If you're craving sugar, reach for some nuts instead of the biscuit tin.

Claim a **FREE** issue of

THE WEEK

Get the week's news in just one hour

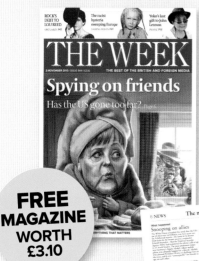

FREE MAGAZINE WORTH £3.10

The Week selects the most important and interesting news stories from the past week and presents them in a fascinating, information-packed magazine. It's easy to read, and after just one hour you are guaranteed to be the most knowledgeable person in the room.

Written for busy people like you, *The Week* is a joy to read, keeping you entertained as well as up to date.

Don't take our word for it. Simply call the number below **and claim your FREE copy today**.

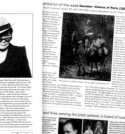

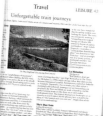

Hydration

There's evidence that as you get older, particularly over 65, thirst sensation diminishes and it's easy to become dehydrated. The best strategy is to keep well hydrated through food and water

Around 70% of your body is made up of water and electrolytes; critical for healthy body function. Water transports nutrients and oxygen around your body, flushes waste products, controls your temperature and aids your digestive system. It's thought that as many as 75% of us are chronically dehydrated and don't drink enough fluid for good health.

Signs of dehydration include tiredness, dark urine, feeling thirsty, constipation, confusion and irritability, poor concentration, dry mouth and dizziness. Being dehydrated by as little at 10% of your body weight can cause symptoms.

TOP UP TIPS

- Drink water regularly, ideally before you are thirsty

- If you have an office job, make sure you have water on your desk

- Eat plenty of fruit and vegetables which have a high water content

- Carry a water bottle with you when you are out and about, especially during warm weather

- Going to the loo every 2-3 hours is an indication you're well hydrated

- As a general rule of thumb, you need to drink around 1500ml of fluid per day; more if you're active, have a high sweat rate or if the weather is hot

- Drinks containing small amounts of caffeine are included in your fluid intake, they don't dehydrate you as once thought. Juice, milk and squash will all add fluid too.

- While thirst is a good indicator of your hydration needs, the key is to drink before thirst. There's evidence that as you get older, particularly over 65, thirst sensation diminishes, which can lead to dehydration.

- Your urine should be pale straw yellow, not clear, nor should it be dark like apple juice or have a strong odour.

Alcohol

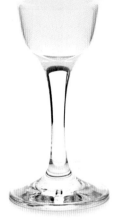

Research has shown that many of us grossly underestimate how much we drink, so what are the facts when it comes to alcohol...

There's nothing wrong with enjoying a drink from time to time, but a recent study has suggested that as many of three quarters of people may be drinking above the recommended daily limit, without even realising it.

The risks

The long-term consequences of high alcohol consumption can be considerable for your health. The risks include liver disease, pancreatitis, diabetes, cancer (especially throat and mouth), heart disease and depression are all increased by just moderate levels of drinking. High alcohol intake can also impair your body's absorption of nutrients from food and bring about vitamin deficiencies.

Is red wine really healthy?

It is thought red wine may have some health benefits in small amounts, but the research is inconclusive and the risks can outweigh the benefits. So get your antioxidants from healthy food instead if you can..

So how much is too much?

Current guidelines recommend that women should not regularly exceed 2-3 units per day, and 3-4 units per day for men, and to have at least one alcohol free day per week.

This may sound reasonable until you start to tot up your intake, as research has shown that most of us underestimate our alcohol intake. Use the www.drinkaware.co.uk unit calculator to work out how much you drink.

What is a unit?

A small (125ml) glass of wine provides around 1.5 units and a pint of beer (at 5% volume) will provide almost 3 units. The average pub/restaurant wine glass is actually 175ml. Some are even 250ml, providing a whopping 3.35 units per glass. Watch out for the percentage strength of wine, as typical measurements are given on 12% volume, which isn't the norm.

Ask yourself...

① How many portions of fruit and veg do you eat?

Current guidelines recommend five portions (a portion is 80g) of fruit and veg per day, although seven to eight is even better. Aim for more vegetables than fruit (ratio 3:2 of vegetables to fruit). Include lots of dark green varieties (rocket, spinach, curly kale, etc) with every meal, and aim for a rainbow of colours. Limit consumption of fruit juice due to high sugar content.

② Do you cut out dairy because it's fattening?

The thinking on dairy is changing. Do you still choose low-fat versions of yoghurt, milk and cheese in a bid to lose weight? Well, the theory on low fat is doing a U-turn. Low-fat dairy will often be more processed, have added sugar or sweetener and won't satiate your appetite. Go for dairy products in their most natural form and choose full-fat milk, cheese and thick, natural yoghurts. Calcium is abundant in dairy produce and it's hard to get enough in your diet without it, so don't cut it out.

③ How much are you drinking?

The culture around alcohol has changed dramatically over the last 20 years. It's now very much part of our lives, widely available and socially acceptable. We use it to unwind after a tough day and to cope with stress. But the majority of people underestimate how much they drink, and many of us are drinking too much without realising.

Check how much you drink at *www.drinkaware.co.uk*

④ Do you cut out carbs to try and lose weight?

The tables are turning on carbs, but they're still the best source of energy, especially for active people, and we need some in our diet to ensure good nutrient and fibre intake. Don't cut them out altogether; just choose foods closest to their natural form. Go for porridge or natural muesli instead of Special K or bran flakes. Rice or potatoes are better than pasta, too. Don't avoid bread altogether, but choose seed-enriched versions and smaller amounts.

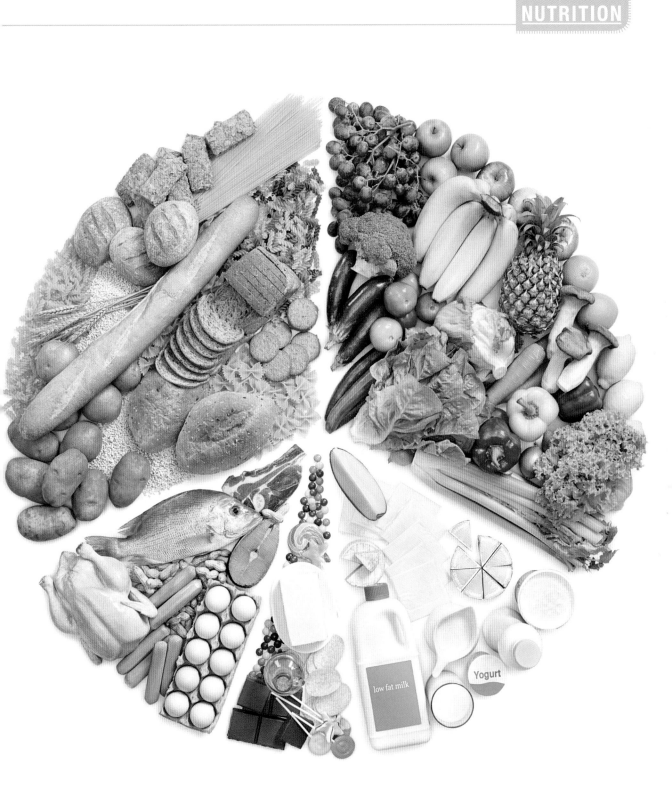

low fat milk

Yogurt

Superfoods

There are healthy foods, and then there are Superfoods. These nutrient packed foods are especially good for our health and some experts claim they can offer protection against conditions such as cancers, heart disease and Alzheimers

Try to include some of these Superfoods in your diet to boost your health and nutrient intake. Here's our pick of the best:

Eggs

The humble egg is one of the most nutritious foods on the planet, providing an excellent source of protein, essential for repair and maintenance of your body. Eggs also contain Vitamin D and A, and essential amino acids. Choose free-range or organic eggs for the best quality. Research has shown that eating eggs for breakfast may help you lose weight, as they help to stabilise your appetite.

Blueberries

The King of all Superfoods, blueberries are packed full of antioxidants, and also high in Vitamin K, potassium and Vitamin C. They are thought to be anti-inflammatory and may reduce your risk of heart disease and cancer. There's even evidence they can help your memory. Frozen berries are just as good as fresh. Eat them fresh or add them to yoghurt, cereal, porridge or smoothies.

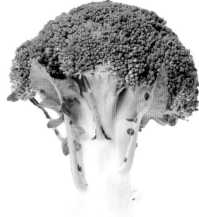

Broccoli

Broccoli is a good source of Vitamin C and folate. It also contains vitamins A and K and is high in fibre, calcium and other antioxidants. Some experts claim it can help combat cancer, high blood pressure, heart disease and diabetes. A recent study showed eating Broccoli may also help in the treatment of arthritis. Try it in soups and stir-fries and different varieties such as purple sprouting broccoli.

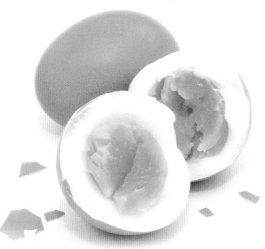

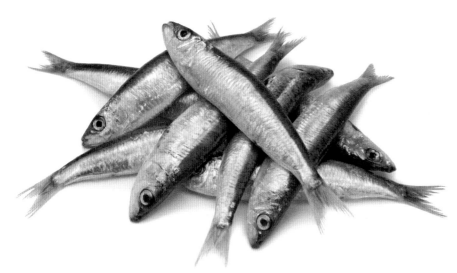

Oily Fish

Fish such as salmon, tuna, mackerel and sardines are packed full of Vitamin D, protein, selenium and a great source of omega-3 fatty acids, a type of fat good for our health. Studies have shown that eating oily fish can lower blood pressure and reduce the risk of heart disease. Evidence strong enough to prompt Government recommendations that we eat at least 2 portions of fish a week. The British Dietetic Association suggest that one of the best things you can do for your heart is to eat oily fish.

Nuts

The health benefits of nuts are indisputable. Rich in calcium, selenium, magnesium and Vitamin E they are also high in fibre and protein and contain important heart-healthy fats. Evidence suggests that eating nuts regularly may reduce the risk of heart disease by as much as 51%. Don't avoid nuts because of the high fat content, they provide vital nutrients and can help stabilise your appetite and balance blood sugar levels. Different nuts are more nutritious than others. Some of the best 'Supernuts' include almonds, brazils and walnuts. Try an organic nut spread instead of butter on your toast.

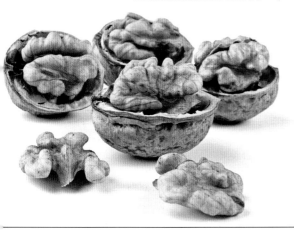

Avocado

The humble avocado contains a rich source of Vitamin E which acts as a powerful antioxidant, reducing your risk of cancer and eye diseases. They are also high in monounsaturated fat, which may help lower LDL cholesterol. In fact, one study found that eating a diet high in avocados significantly lowered LDL cholesterol after just one week. Try adding to salads or mashing into sandwiches.

It's easy to include Superfoods in your diet. Try out some of our delicious 'Superfood Recipes' over the next few pages: ◗

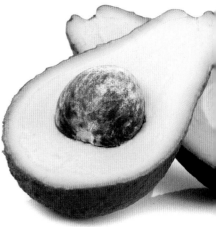

Roasted Squash Superfood Salad

with pumpkin seeds, chilli and feta cheese

INGREDIENTS

serves 4

1 small 'queen' squash

50g pumpkin seeds

1 tbsp olive oil

100g rocket leaves or similar

Sea salt and freshly ground black pepper

½ tsp cumin seeds, crushed

1 small red chill, seeds removed and chopped

100g feta cheese

2 tbsp fresh coriander leaves, chopped

1 tbsp white balsamic wine vinegar

2 tbsp extra virgin olive oil or pumpkin seed oil

METHOD

① Heat the oven to 200°C/400°F/gas mark 6.

② Peel the squash, cut it in half and scoop out the seeds. Cut it into wedges. Place in a bowl, drizzle over the oil and shake around so that they're well coated. Lay the wedges onto a baking tray, sprinkle with a large pinch of sea salt and ground pepper, and the crushed cumin seeds. Roast for about 25 minutes, until soft and slightly caramelised. Remove from the oven and leave to cool.

③ Reduce the oven temperature to 160°C/325°F/gas mark 3. Roast the pumpkin seeds on a flat baking sheet for five minutes. Remove from the oven and cool.

④ Arrange the salad leaves on a large, flat serving dish. Lay the squash slices on top and scatter with the pumpkin seeds, feta cheese, red chilli and coriander leaves. Whisk together the oil and vinegar with a pinch of sea salt and drizzle over the salad just before serving.

NUTRITION PER SERVING
ENERGY (KCAL) 305
PROTEIN (G) 9
CARBOHYDRATE (G) 23
FAT (G) 22 OF WHICH
SUGARS (G) 6 OF WHICH
SATURATES (G) 6 SALT (G) 1
FIBRE (G) 1

WHY IT'S GOOD FOR YOU

▶ **Well-balanced salad with slow-burning carbohydrate, protein and healthy omega 3 fats.**

▶ **Rich in vitamins A, C, D, B6, B12, K and E, and minerals such as calcium, iron, sodium, magnesium, potassium, and fibre.**

▶ **Energy-boosting superfood phytochemicals, immune-supporting antioxidants to help reduce the risk of cancers, stroke and cardiovascular disease.**

▶ **Anti-inflammatory properties from the chilli, ginger and squash.**

RECIPE COURTESY OF KATE PERCY, AUTHOR OF *GO FASTER FOOD* AND *GO FASTER FOOD FOR KIDS* AVAILABLE ON AMAZON.CO.UK OR AT WWW.GOFASTERFOOD.COM.

Spanish Almond & Orange Cake

Based on the Tarta di Santiago, this deliciously light cake has just three basic ingredients: almonds, sugar and eggs

INGREDIENTS
serves 6-8

4 large, free-range eggs, separated

Zest of 1 large orange

225g caster sugar

225g ground almonds

½ tsp cinnamon

1 tbsp freshly squeezed orange juice

Icing sugar to decorate

METHOD

❶ Preheat the oven to 180°C/350°F/gas mark 4.

❷ Lightly grease a 23cm springform cake tin or flan dish with butter.

❸ Whisk the egg whites to soft peak stage with an electric whisk.

❹ Put the egg yolks, orange zest and sugar into a separate bowl, and whisk until pale and creamy. Stir in the almonds, the cinnamon and the orange juice.

❺ Fold in the egg whites, a little at a time.

❻ Pour the mixture into the cake tin and cook in the oven for about 30–35 minutes, until golden. If you poke a skewer into the middle of the cake, it should come out clean. Cool in the tin, on a wire rack.

❼ When cool, decorate with icing sugar. Enjoy with a dollop of natural yoghurt or crème fraîche.

WHY IT'S GOOD FOR YOU

▶ A natural energy food; moist, gluten-free and light on the stomach.

▶ Rich in cholesterol-reducing, heart-healthy mono-unsaturated fats. Almonds contain a double-barreled protection against cardiovascular disease and diabetes. Low in GI, they help control blood sugar levels and lower cholesterol.

▶ Packed with good-quality carbohydrate and protein.

▶ Contains magnesium, important for energy production and bone health, and potassium, which helps control blood pressure.

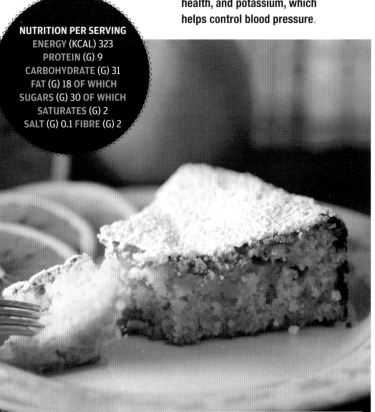

NUTRITION PER SERVING
ENERGY (KCAL) 323
PROTEIN (G) 9
CARBOHYDRATE (G) 31
FAT (G) 18 OF WHICH
SUGARS (G) 30 OF WHICH
SATURATES (G) 2
SALT (G) 0.1 FIBRE (G) 2

Go Faster Rainbow Breakfast Crunch

This tasty recipe gives you more granola than you'll need; keep the rest in an airtight container

INGREDIENTS

200g unrefined whole rolled porridge oats

250g mixed nuts and seeds (flaked almonds, sunflower and pumpkin seeds, walnuts, pistachios, pecans and hazelnuts)

½ tsp cinnamon

½ tsp ground ginger

2 tbsp honey or maple syrup

2 tbsp sunflower oil

2 tbsp water

100g mixed dried fruit (raisins, crystallised ginger, dried apricots, figs and/or dates), chopped (optional)

250g natural yoghurt

100g soft berry fruit (blackberries, blackcurrants, blueberries, raspberries or strawberries)

1 tsp sugar

METHOD

1 Preheat the oven to 180°C/350°F/gas mark 4.

2 To make the granola, mix together the oats, nuts and seeds with the cinnamon, ginger, honey, oil and water. Spread the mixture evenly onto a large baking sheet.

3 Bake for 20 minutes until golden, turning the mixture after 10 minutes for it to brown evenly. Leave to cool for five minutes or so. It will crisp up like magic.

4 Add the dried fruit if using.

5 Put the soft fruit in a bowl and sprinkle over the sugar.

6 In a tall sundae dish or glass, carefully arrange the yoghurt, granola and fruit in layers, to create colourful stripes. Serve immediately.

WHY IT'S GOOD FOR YOU

▶ **Well-balanced with slow-burning carbohydrate, protein and healthy omega 3 fats.**

▶ **A rainbow selection of superfood phytochemicals, including flavonoids, anthocyanins and ellagic acid, antioxidants to help reduce the risk of cancers, Alzheimer's and diabetes.**

▶ **Rich in vitamins and minerals such as potassium, calcium iron and fibre.**

▶ **Contributes to strong bones, healthy heart, brain and immune system.**

▶ **Quick and easy to prepare.**

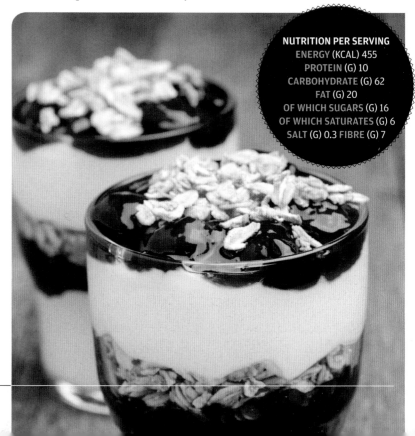

NUTRITION PER SERVING
ENERGY (KCAL) 455
PROTEIN (G) 10
CARBOHYDRATE (G) 62
FAT (G) 20
OF WHICH SUGARS (G) 16
OF WHICH SATURATES (G) 6
SALT (G) 0.3 FIBRE (G) 7

RECIPE COURTESY OF KATE PERCY, AUTHOR OF GO FASTER FOOD AND GO FASTER FOOD FOR KIDS AVAILABLE ON AMAZON.CO.UK OR AT WWW.GOFASTERFOOD.COM.

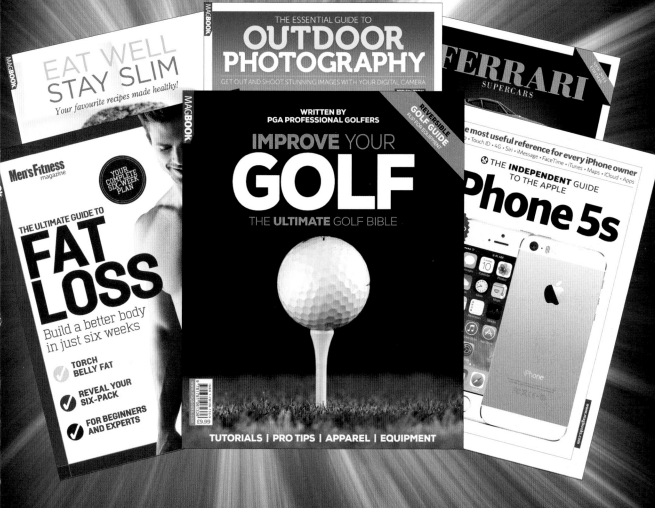

Warm Salad of Seared Tuna

with white beans

INGREDIENTS

serves 2

50g pancetta cubes

1 tbsp olive oil

1 clove garlic, peeled and crushed

400g can of butter beans

2 semi-dried/sunblush tomatoes, chopped

1 tbsp lemon juice

Large handful flat-leaf parsley, chopped

1 tbsp balsamic vinegar

2 tbsp extra virgin olive oil

1 preserved lemon, sliced very finely, pulp removed, plus a little of the brine for the dressing

Bunch of rocket and/or spinach

Salt and freshly ground black pepper to taste

2 thick tuna steaks

METHOD

❶ Sauté the pancetta gently in a tbsp of the olive oil for five minutes until cooked. Add the garlic, white beans, tomatoes, lemon juice and half of the parsley, and heat through. Season with salt and pepper.

❷ Make the dressing by mixing together the balsamic vinegar, 2 tbsp of extra virgin olive oil, the preserved lemon, the rest of the parsley, salt, pepper and a few drops of the preserved lemon brine. Arrange the rocket and/or spinach on two plates and spoon on the white bean mixture.

❸ Lightly brush the tuna with a little olive oil and heat the griddle pan or frying pan to very hot. Fry the steaks for a couple of minutes on each side. Don't overcook the tuna, or it will go rubbery! It should be pink inside and will continue to cook slightly after you've removed it from the pan.

❹ Place a steak on top of each bed of white beans and generously drizzle over the dressing.

NUTRITION PER SERVING
ENERGY (KCAL) 509
PROTEIN (G) 35
CARBOHYDRATE (G) 20
FAT (G) 33 OF WHICH
SUGARS (G) 2 OF WHICH
SATURATES (G) 7
SALT (G) 2.5 FIBRE (G) 4

WHY IT'S GOOD FOR YOU

▶ **Well-balanced meal with low GI, sustaining carbohydrate, quality protein and heart-healthy omega 3 fats.**

▶ **Rich in vitamins and minerals such as potassium, calcium iron and fibre.**

▶ **Contributes to strong bones, healthy heart, brain and immune system.**

▶ **Energy-boosting, and quick and easy to prepare.**

RECIPE COURTESY OF KATE PERCY, AUTHOR OF *GO FASTER FOOD* AND *GO FASTER FOOD FOR KIDS* AVAILABLE ON AMAZON.CO.UK OR AT WWW.GOFASTERFOOD.COM.

Sweet Potato & Chickpea Soup

with coconut oil

INGREDIENTS

serves 4

2 tbsp coconut oil

1 onion, finely sliced

2 sweet potatoes, or 1 large one, peeled and cut into small cubes

2 x garlic cloves, crushed

2 cm chunk root ginger, grated

1 tsp cumin seeds, dry fried for one minute and crushed in pestle and mortar

½ tsp cinnamon

¼ tsp cayenne pepper

¼ tsp English mustard powder

1 x 400g can chickpeas

2 x tomatoes or 100ml passata

1 tsp honey

1 litre vegetable or chicken stock

Salt and freshly ground black pepper to taste

METHOD

1 Heat the oil in a large saucepan and gently fry the onion for a few minutes.

2 Add the sweet potato, the garlic and the ginger and fry for a further minute or two. Add the cumin, cinnamon, cayenne and mustard powder, and cook for 30 seconds, gently stirring the mixture all the time.

3 Stir in the chickpeas, the tomatoes and the honey, and cook for two minutes, stirring frequently. Add the stock and bring the mixture to the boil. Cover and simmer for 10 minutes until the sweet potato is tender.

4 Purée the soup in a blender until smooth. Season with plenty of salt and black pepper.

NUTRITION PER SERVING

ENERGY (KCAL) 258
PROTEIN (G) 10
CARBOHYDRATE (G) 36
FAT (G) 9
OF WHICH SUGARS (G) 10
OF WHICH SATURATES (G) 1
SALT (G) 1.5 FIBRE (G) 7

WHY IT'S GOOD FOR YOU

▶ **Coconut oil has many health-giving qualities: it has antiviral, antibiotic and antifungal properties, can help burn fat more efficiently and contribute to better brain function.**

▶ **Chickpeas provide a source of protein, plus minerals and fibre.**

▶ **Anti-inflammatory properties from the ginger and the spices.**

▶ **Energy-boosting superfood phytochemicals in the sweet potato, and immune-supporting antioxidants to help reduce the risk of cancers, stroke and cardiovascular disease.**

Nutrition round-up

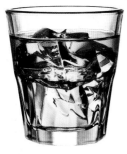

There's growing evidence that people aged between 65 and 90 are drinking at harmful levels, but fail to realise the damaging effects on their health, as they don't consider themselves to be heavy drinkers. Keep a track of your alcohol intake at *www.drinkaware.co.uk*.

"If you really want to lose weight and keep it off, there's a lot more to it than just what you eat. My advice would be not to do what everyone else is doing, or follow the current trendy diet, but to work out your own path, and find a system that works for you."

LIFE COACH PETE COHEN

75% of us don't get enough magnesium in our diet. Stress, raised cortisol levels, processed food, caffeine and alcohol can all lower your levels of magnesium, and we also lose significant amounts through sweat loss.

"Do you suffer from painful joints? If so, you may need a good oiling! A daily handful of walnuts, and oily fish three times a week will keep your joints supple and pain free."

MIGUEL TORIBIO-MATEAS

CALCIUM IS THE MOST ABUNDANT MINERAL

in your body and vital for strong bones and teeth. If you don't get enough calcium, you can risk health problems related to weak bones. Bone loss can affect people over 50, especially post-menopausal women, where bone is lost more quickly than it's formed.

There's evidence that as you get older, particularly over 65, thirst sensation diminishes and it's easy to become dehydrated. The best strategy is to keep well hydrated through food and water.

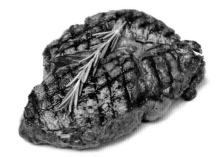

A RECENT ARTICLE BY CARDIOLOGIST DR ASEEM MALHOTRA, published in the *British Medical Journal* in October 2013, suggested that saturated fat – found in foods such as butter, cheese and red meat – may not be as bad for us as previously thought.